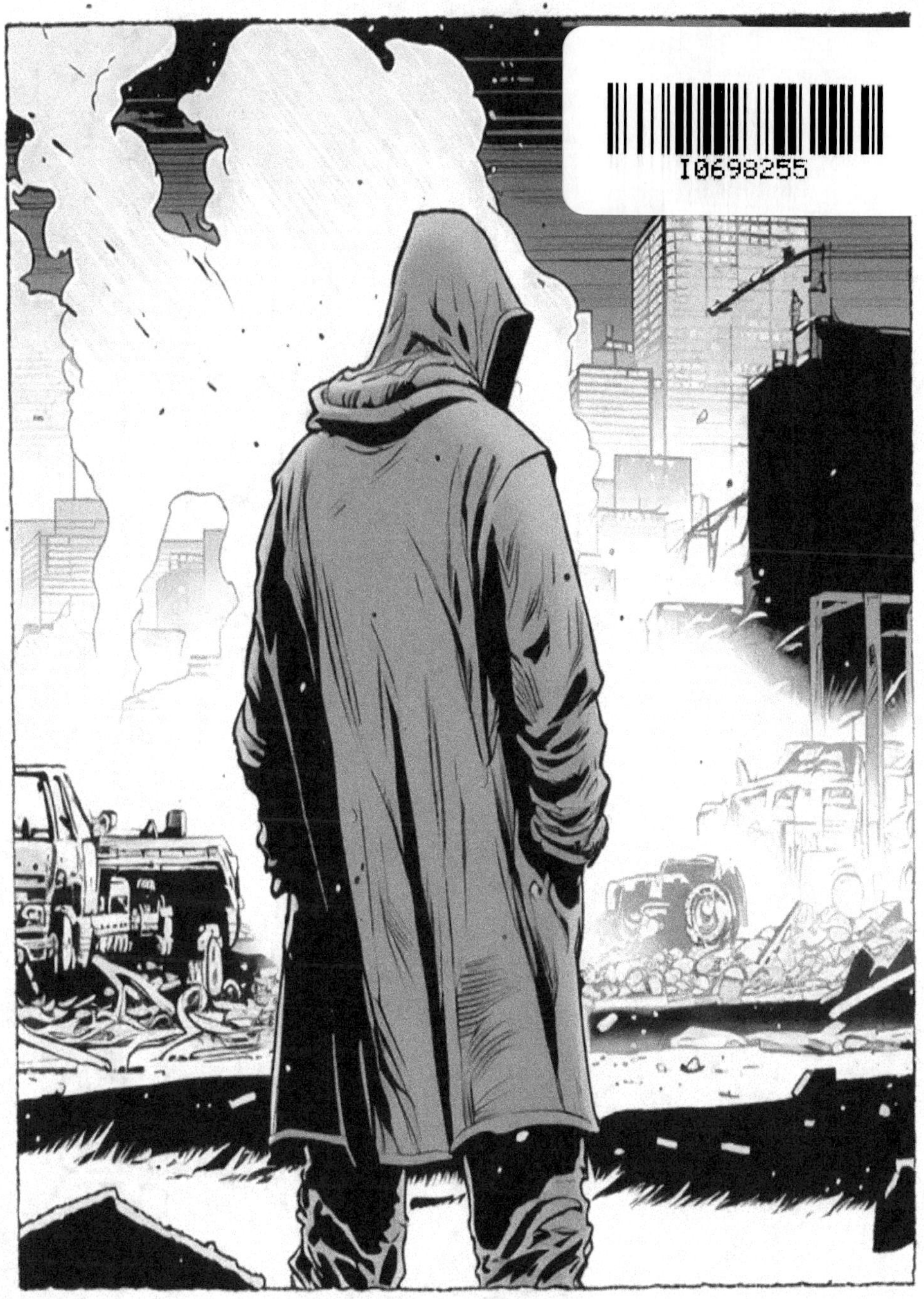

FIGHTING AGAINST THE POISONOUS FOOD INDUSTRY.

Book Chapters:

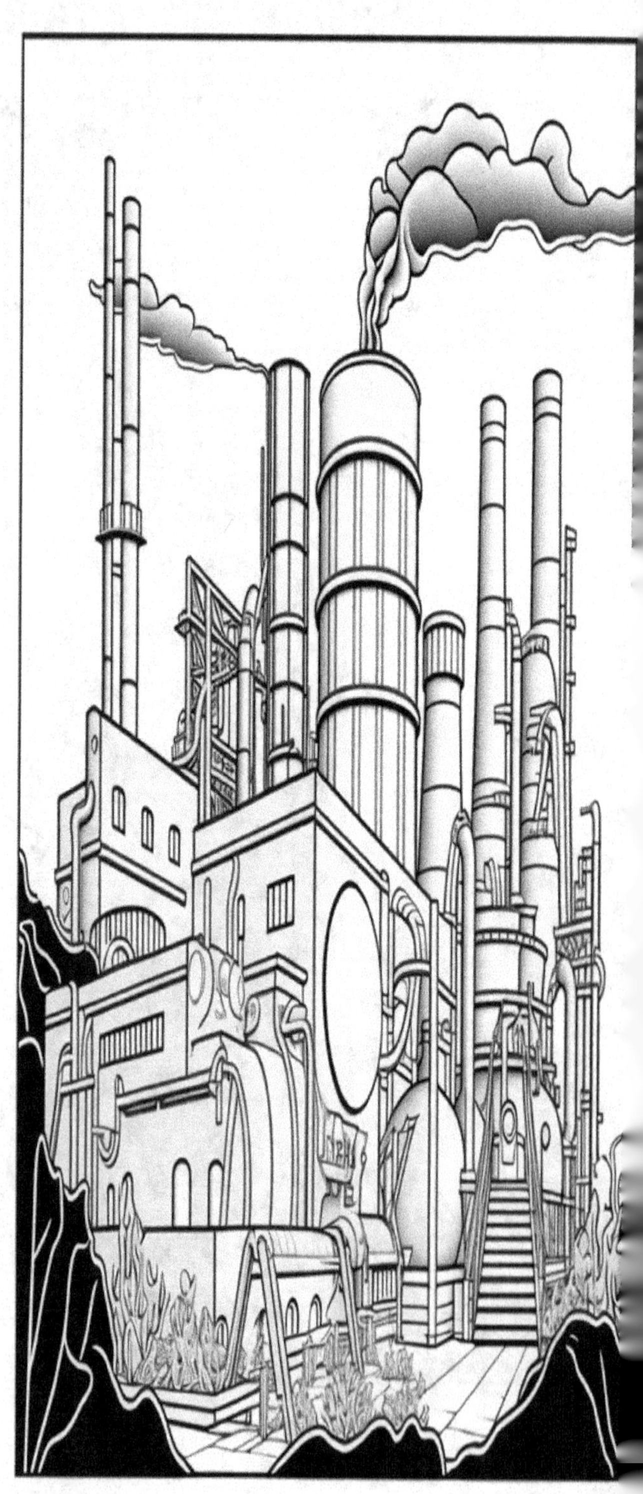

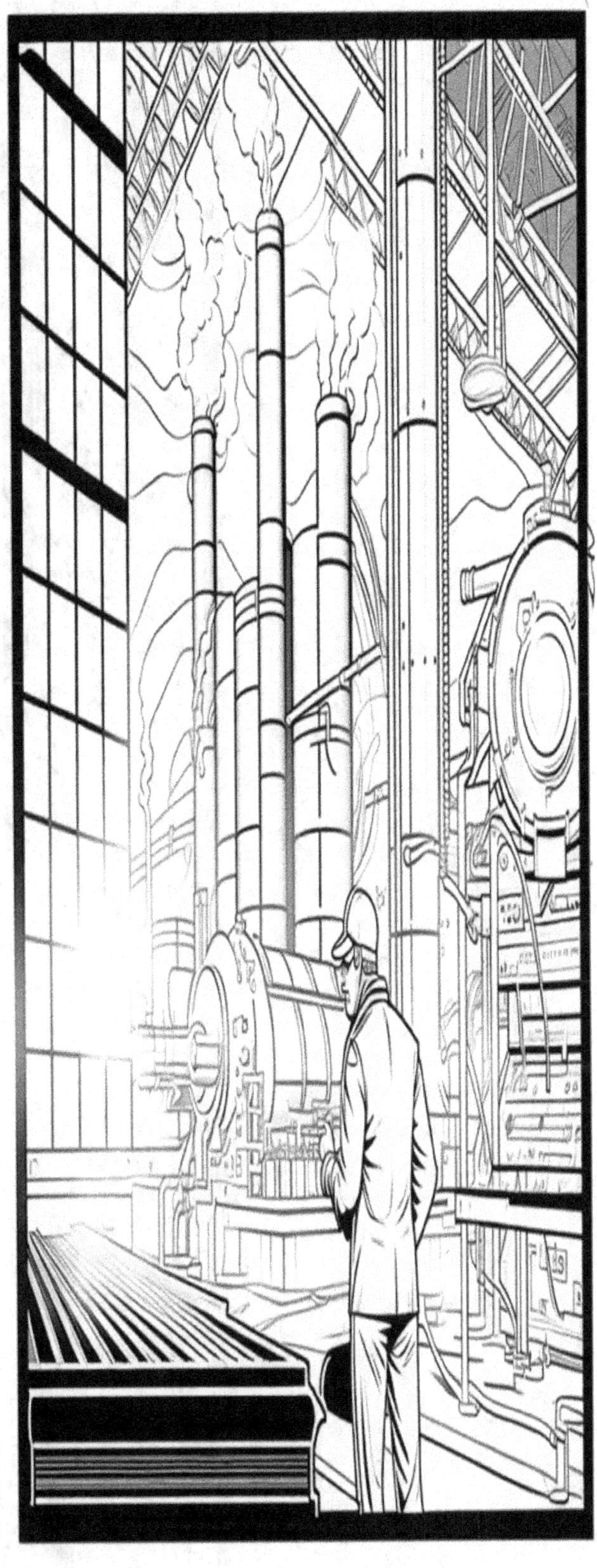

15. Conclusion: The Future of Microgreens and Your Role in It

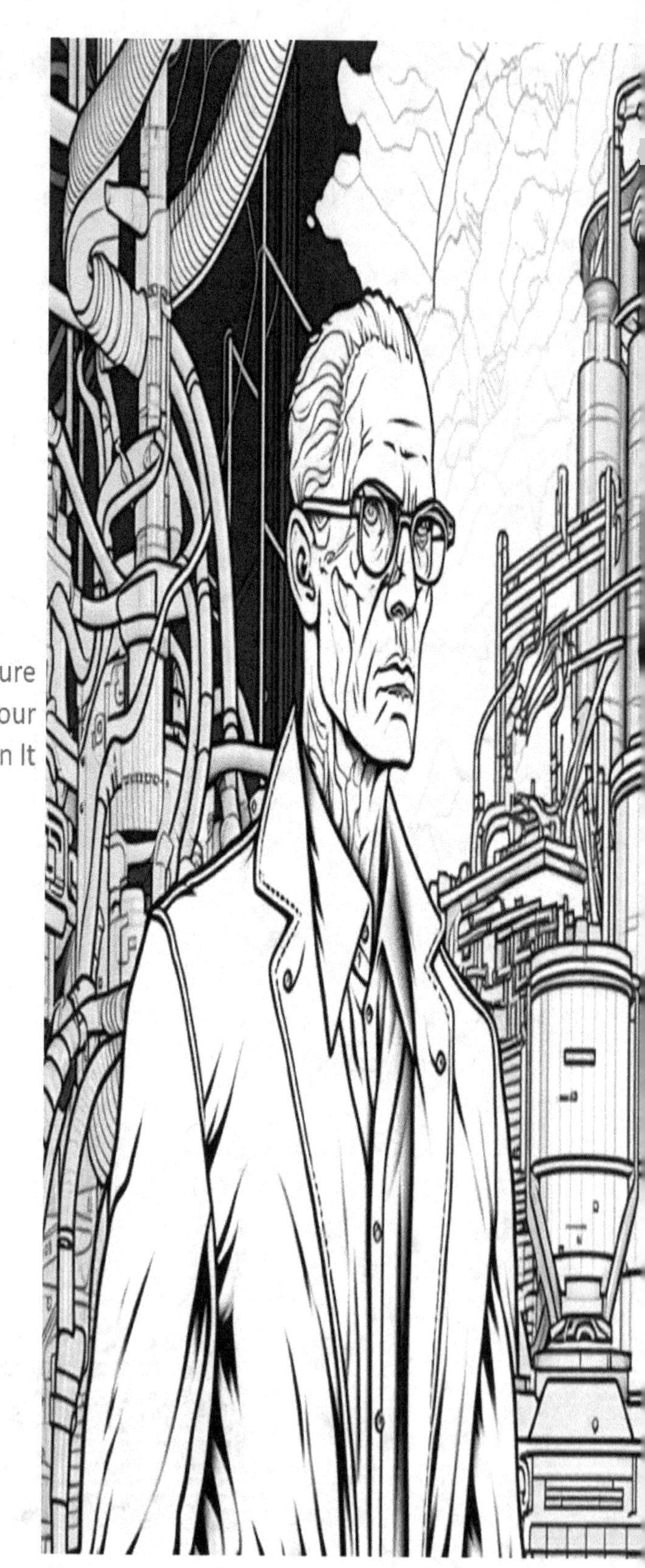

INTRO

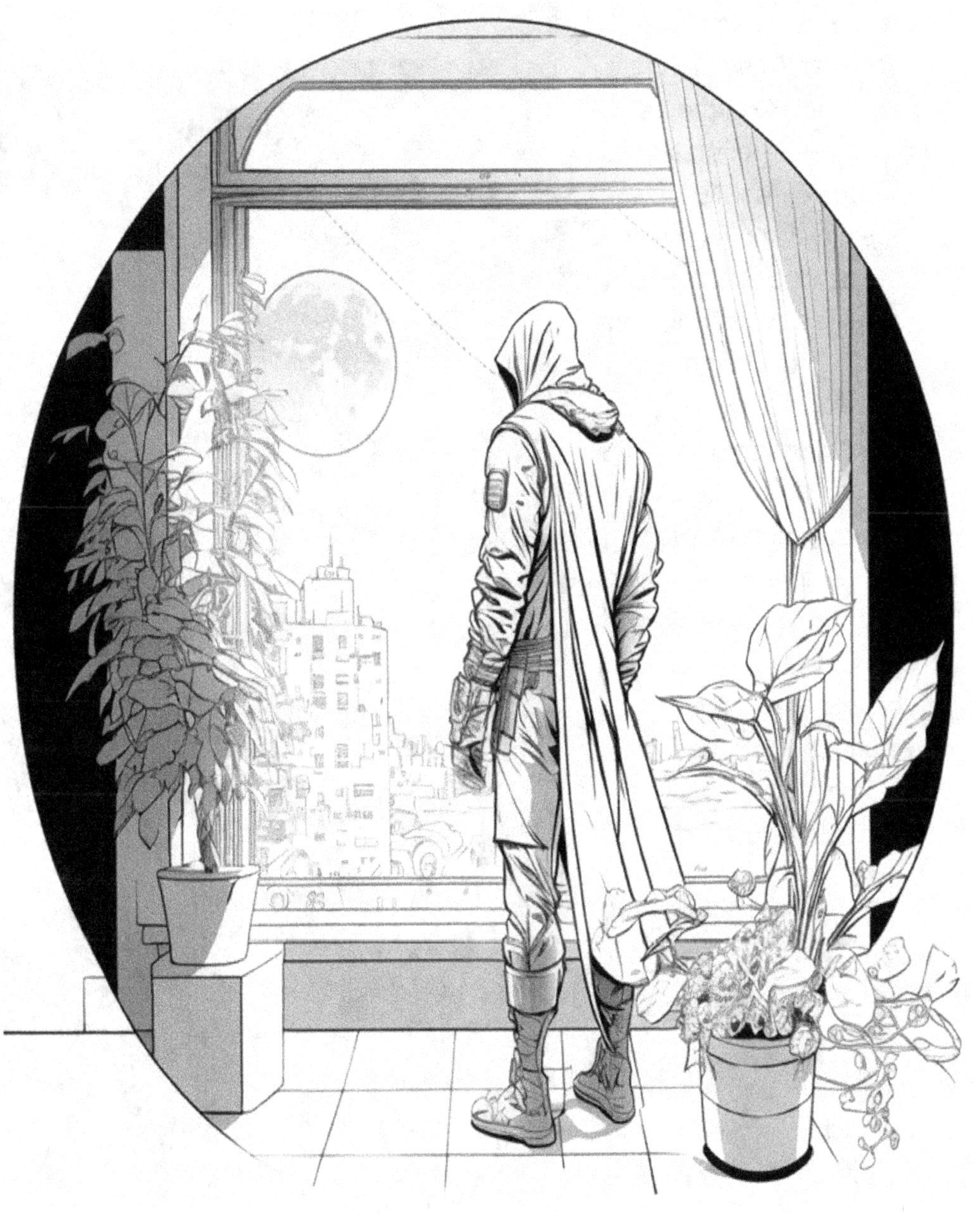

At one point or another, we have all heard the saying, "You are what you eat." Unfortunately, in today's world, this statement could not be any more accurate. With the rise of processed foods, genetically modified organisms (GMOs), and chemicals in our food, it is no surprise that many people are suffering from chronic illnesses.

Grocery stores are filled with products that are marketed as healthy, yet contain a vast array of additives, preservatives, and chemicals. These chemicals are used to enhance flavor, extend shelf life, and make the food more visually appealing. However, what most people do not know is that these chemicals can have detrimental effects on our health.

Let's take a closer look at some of the chemicals found in grocery food and how they can affect our health:

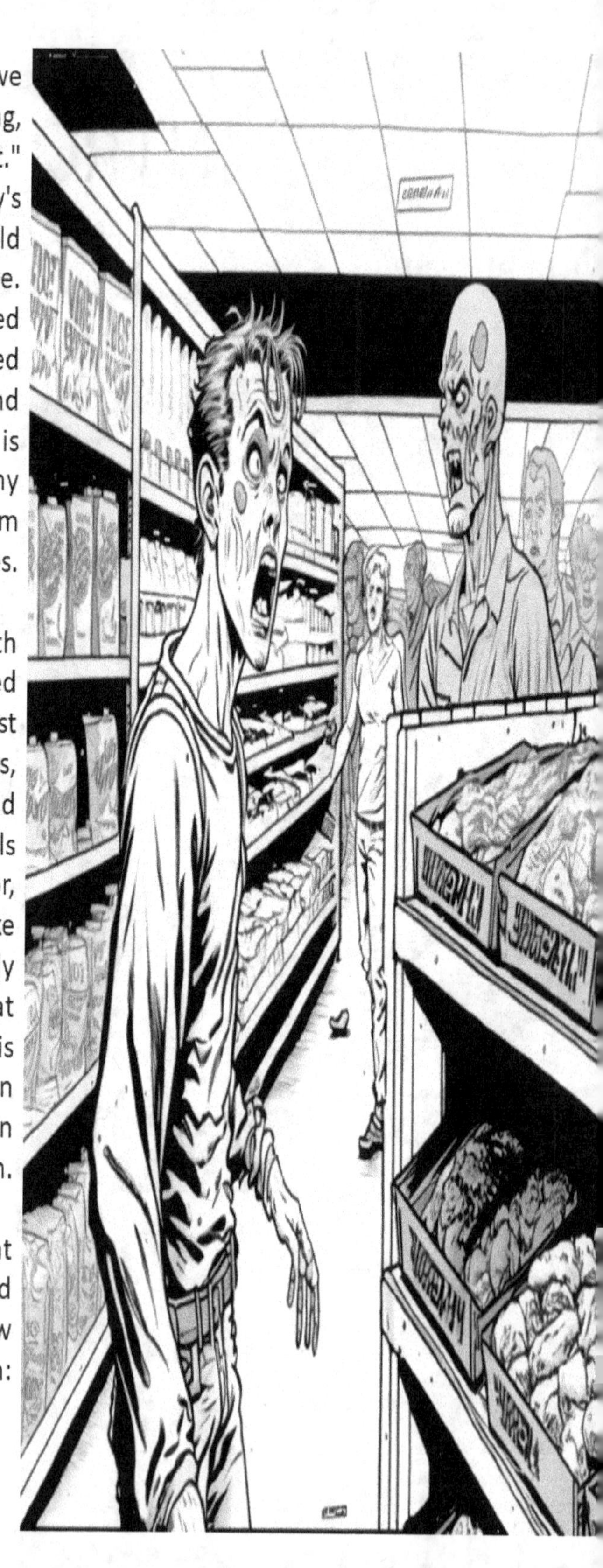

Artificial Sweeteners

Artificial sweeteners are commonly used in many processed foods and beverages. These sweeteners, such as aspartame and sucralose, are often marketed as a healthy alternative to sugar. However, these sweeteners have been linked to a variety of health problems, including headaches, digestive issues, and even cancer.

Trans Fats

Trans fats are commonly found in processed foods, such as fried foods, margarine, and baked goods. These fats have been linked to an increased risk of heart disease, stroke, and diabetes.

MSG

Monosodium glutamate (MSG) is a flavor enhancer commonly found in processed foods, such as chips, soups, and frozen dinners. MSG has been linked to a variety of health problems, including

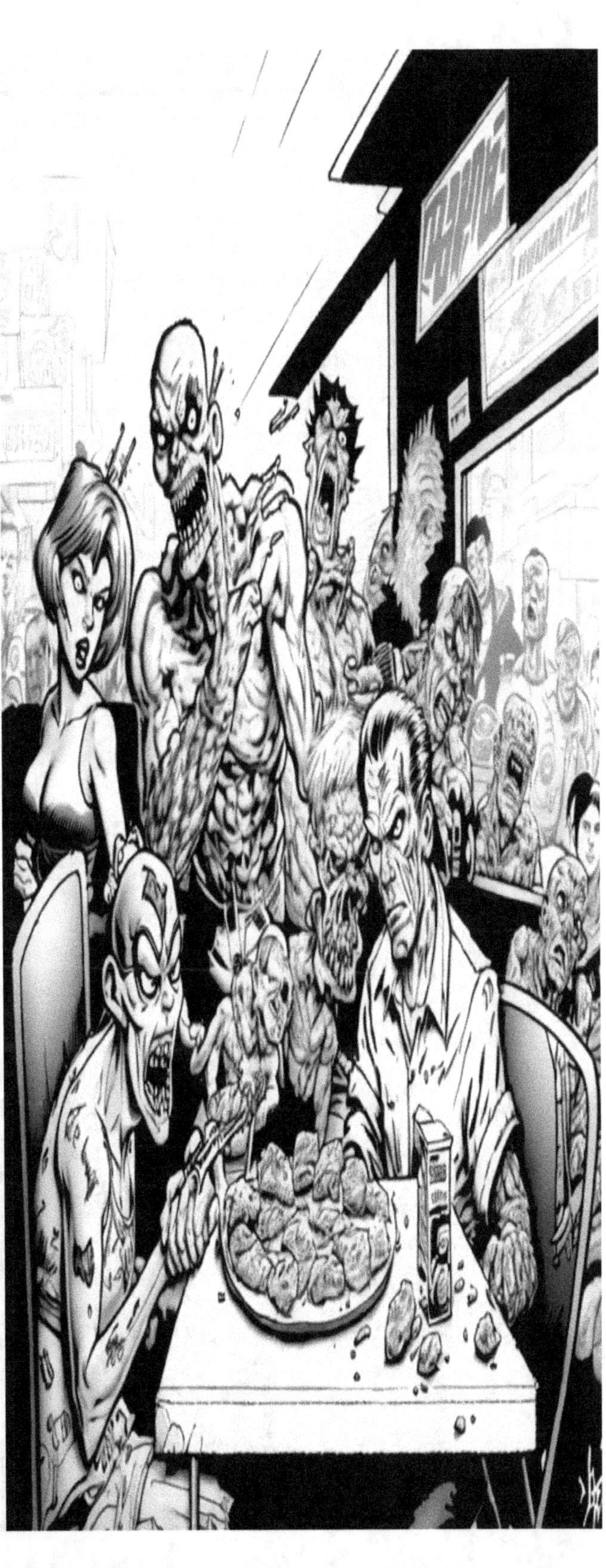

headaches, nausea, and even brain damage.

High Fructose Corn Syrup (HFCS)

HFCS is a sweetener commonly found in processed foods, such as soda, candy, and baked goods. This sweetener has been linked to an increased risk of obesity, type 2 diabetes, and heart disease.

Pesticides

Pesticides are commonly used in conventionally grown fruits and vegetables to prevent pests from damaging crops. However, these chemicals can also harm humans. Exposure to pesticides has been linked to an increased risk of cancer, birth defects, and neurological problems.

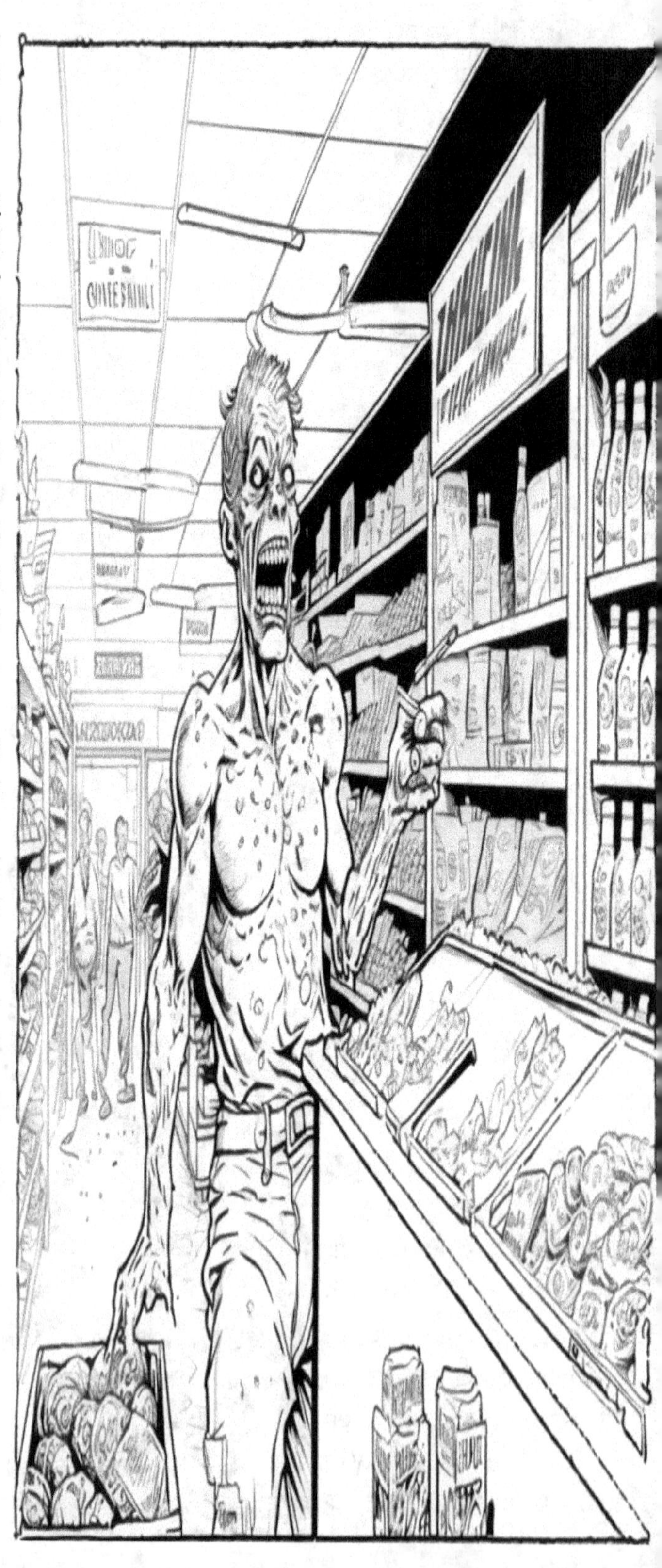

Artificial Colors and Flavors

Artificial colors and flavors are commonly added to processed foods to enhance their appearance and taste. However, these additives have been linked to a variety of health problems, including hyperactivity in children and allergic reactions.

What Can You Do?

It is essential to be aware of the chemicals in your food and make informed decisions when purchasing groceries. One way to do this is to choose organic, non-GMO, and whole foods. These foods are free from harmful chemicals and are packed with nutrients that your body needs to thrive.

Another way to reduce your exposure to harmful chemicals is to cook your food at home using fresh ingredients.

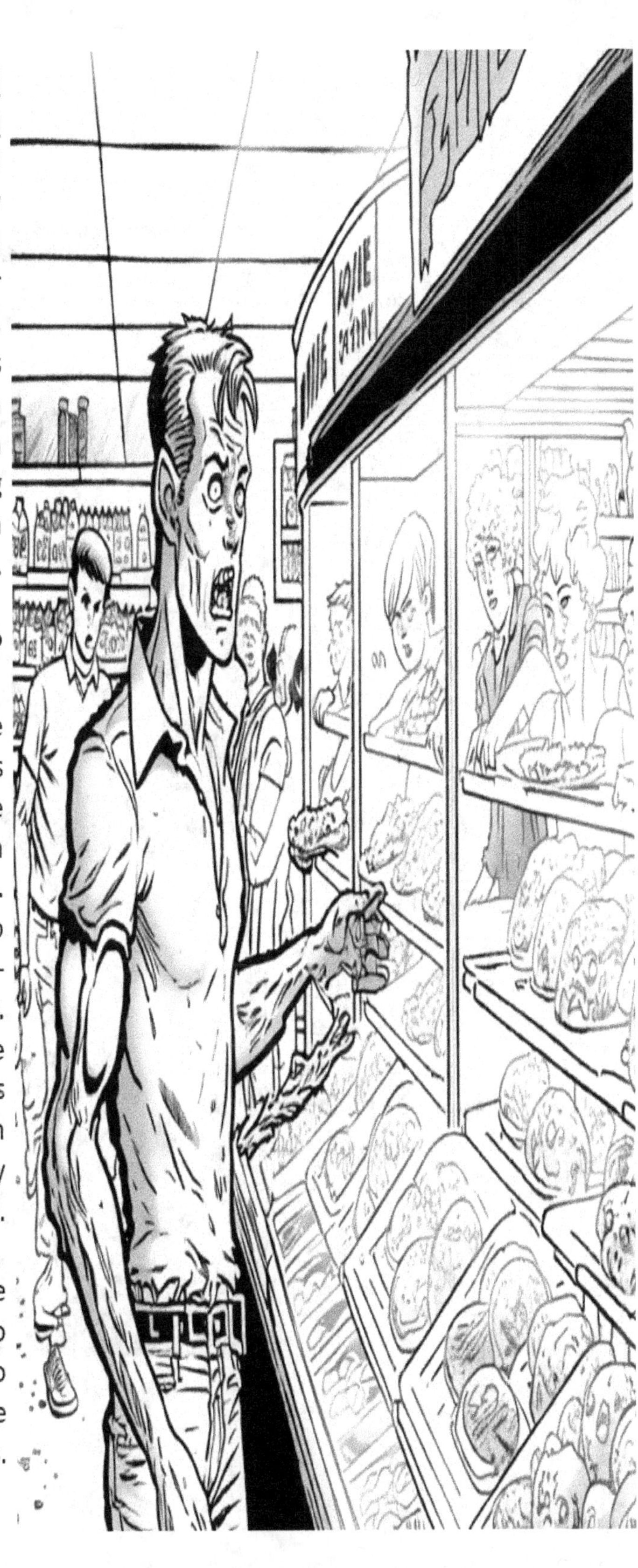

By doing so, you can control the ingredients that go into your meals and ensure that you are eating a healthy, balanced diet.

In Conclusion

The chemicals found in grocery food can have detrimental effects on our health. It is essential to be aware of these chemicals and make informed decisions when purchasing groceries. By choosing organic, non-GMO, and whole foods and cooking at home using fresh ingredients, you can reduce your exposure to harmful chemicals and improve your overall health.

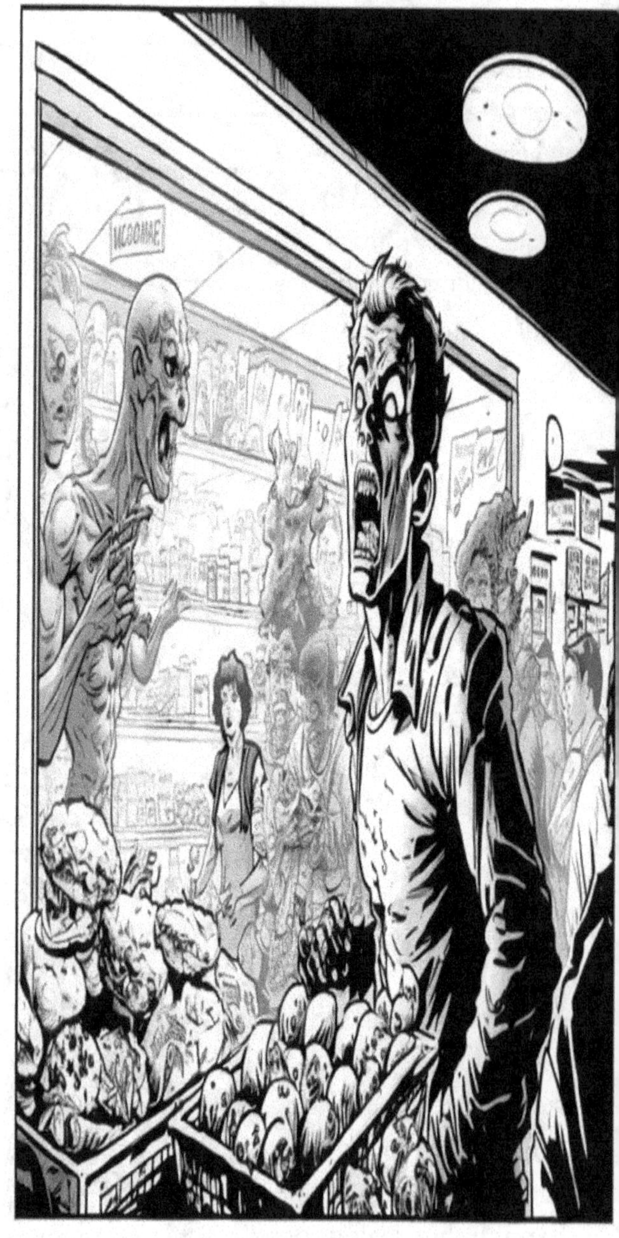

CHAPTER 1: INTRODUCTION TO MICROGREENS: WHAT ARE THEY AND WHY SHOULD YOU GROW THEM?

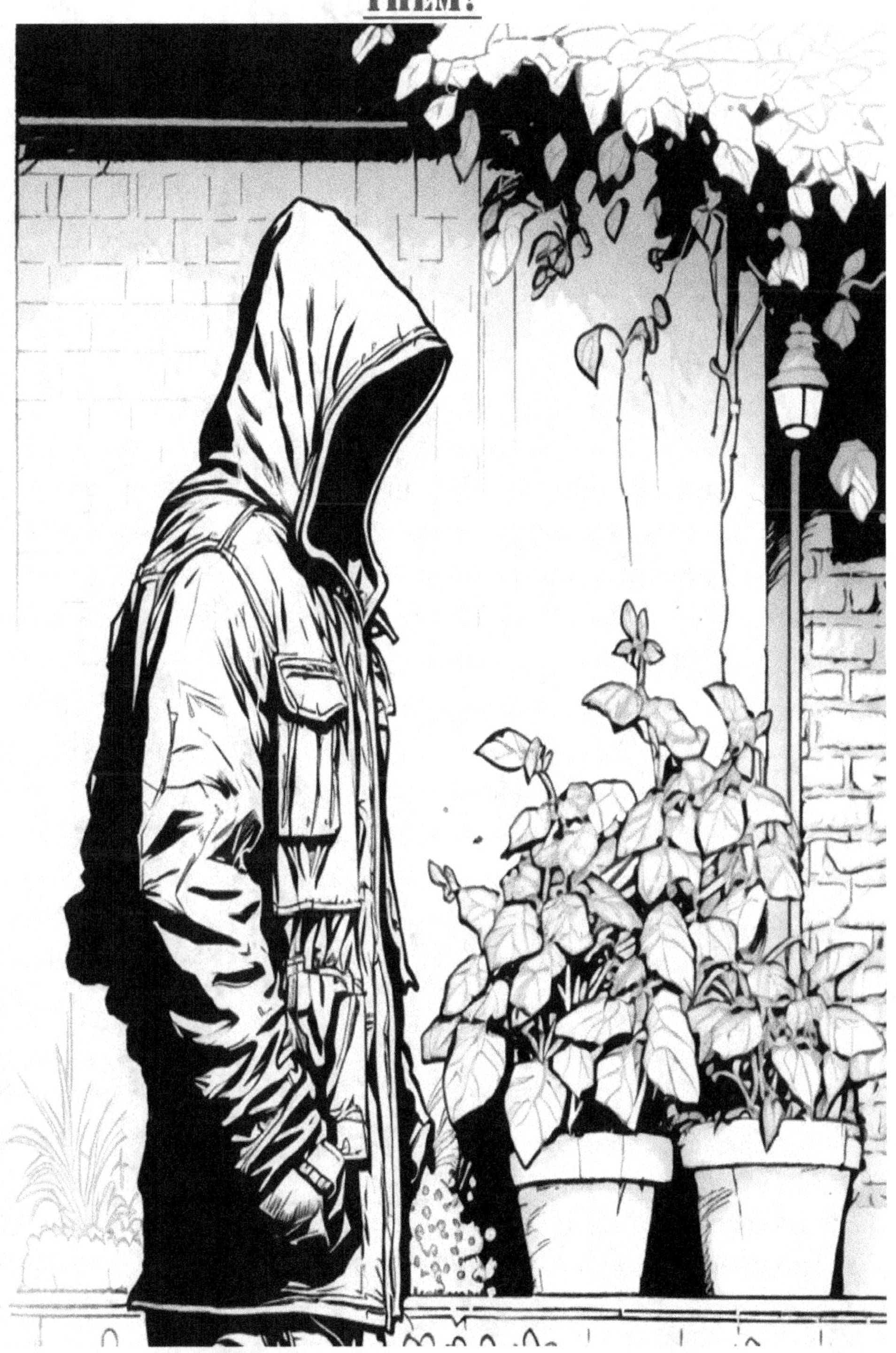

Microgreens are tiny plants that are harvested when they are just a few inches tall, usually within 10-14 days of germination. They are packed with nutrients, including vitamins C, E, and K, as well as iron, calcium, and antioxidants. Some studies have even shown that microgreens contain higher levels of these nutrients than their fully grown counterparts.

Not only are microgreens nutritious, but they are also easy to grow and can be grown year-round, making them an excellent addition to any diet. They can be grown in small spaces, such as apartments or houses, and can be harvested in as little as two weeks. Plus, growing your own microgreens is a fun and rewarding way to engage with nature and promote healthy eating habits.

So why should you grow microgreens? For starters, they are a great way to add fresh greens to your meals without having to worry

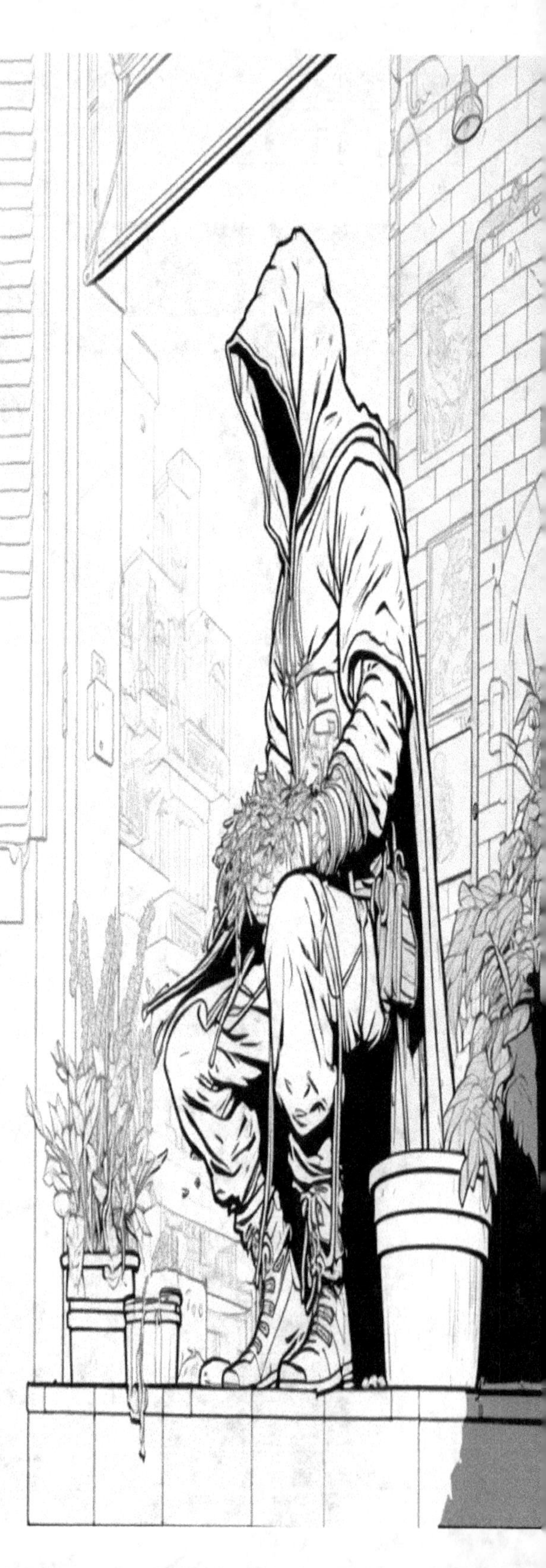

about pesticides or other harmful chemicals. They are also more sustainable than buying pre-packaged greens from the grocery store, as they require less water and transportation. Plus, growing your own microgreens is a great way to save money on groceries and reduce food waste, as you can harvest only what you need for each meal.

Overall, microgreens are a nutritious and sustainable addition to any diet, and growing your own microgreen garden is a fun and rewarding way to promote healthy eating

microgreens are also environmentally friendly. They require less water, fertilizer, and space than traditional gardening, and they can be grown year-round, reducing the need for transportation and storage of produce.

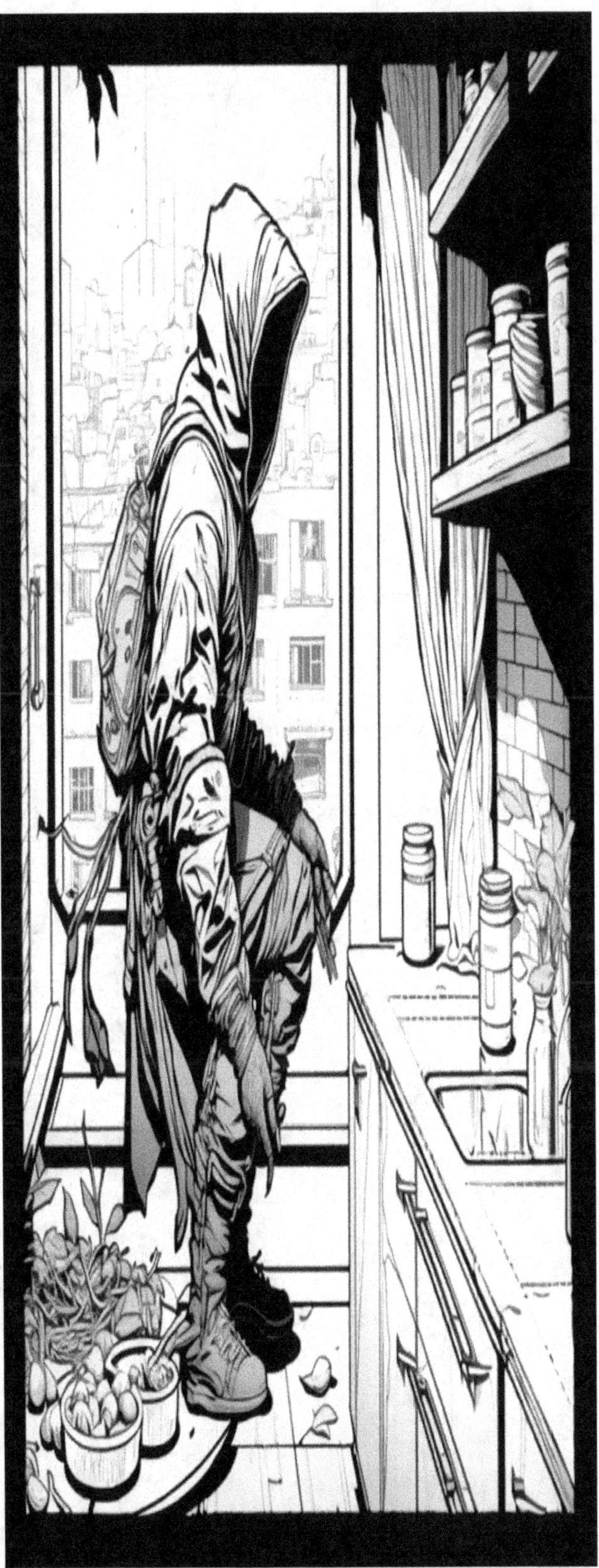

Microgreens are also economical. They can be grown from relatively inexpensive seeds, and they can be harvested multiple times, increasing the yield and reducing waste. Plus, by growing your own microgreens, you can save money on expensive store-bought greens and reduce your grocery bill.

Overall, microgreens are a versatile and nutritious addition to any diet and growing them at home is a fun and rewarding hobby. In the following chapters, we will explore the benefits of growing microgreens in more detail and provide you with all the information you need to start your own microgreen garden.

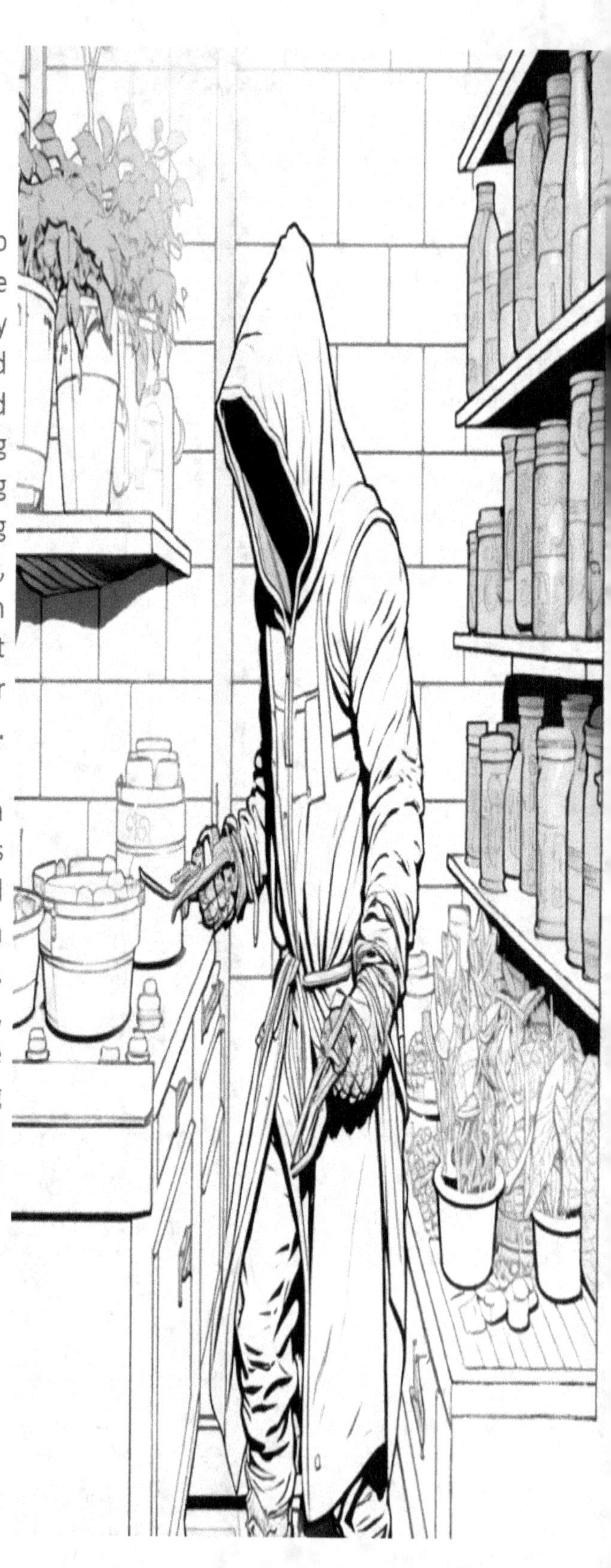

CHAPTER 2. THE BENEFITS OF MICROGREENS: NUTRITIONAL AND ENVIRONMENTAL

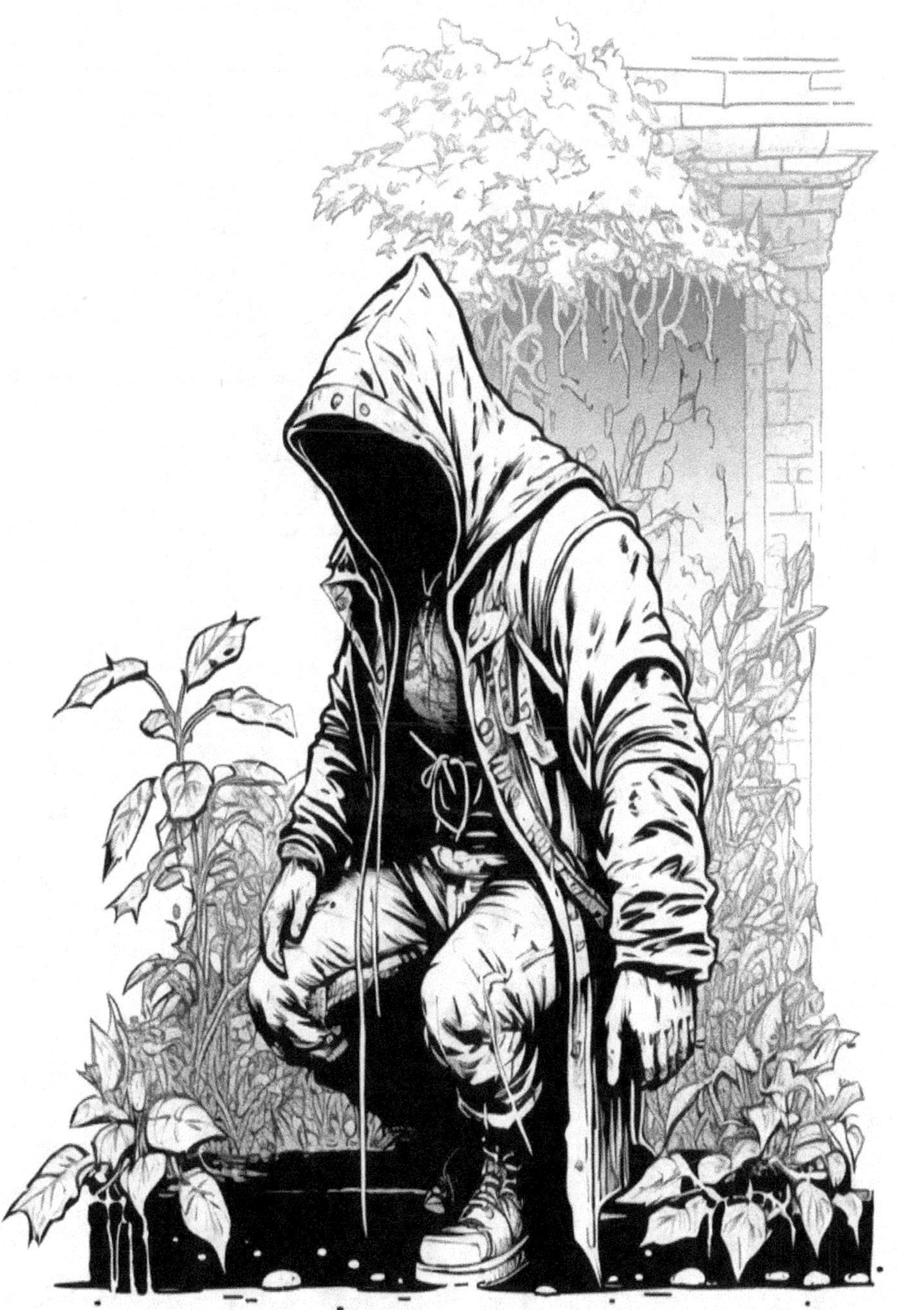

Microgreens are not only delicious, but they also offer a variety of health benefits. Because they are harvested at an early stage of growth, microgreens contain higher levels of nutrients than their mature counterparts. In fact, some studies have shown that microgreens can contain up to 40 times more nutrients than fully grown plants!

Microgreens are also packed with antioxidants, which help protect your cells from damage caused by free radicals. They are a good source of fiber, which promotes digestive health, and they contain enzymes that aid in digestion and nutrient absorption.
In addition to their health benefits, growing microgreens is also good for the environment. By growing your own food, you can reduce your carbon footprint and help to minimize the impact of transportation and storage of produce.

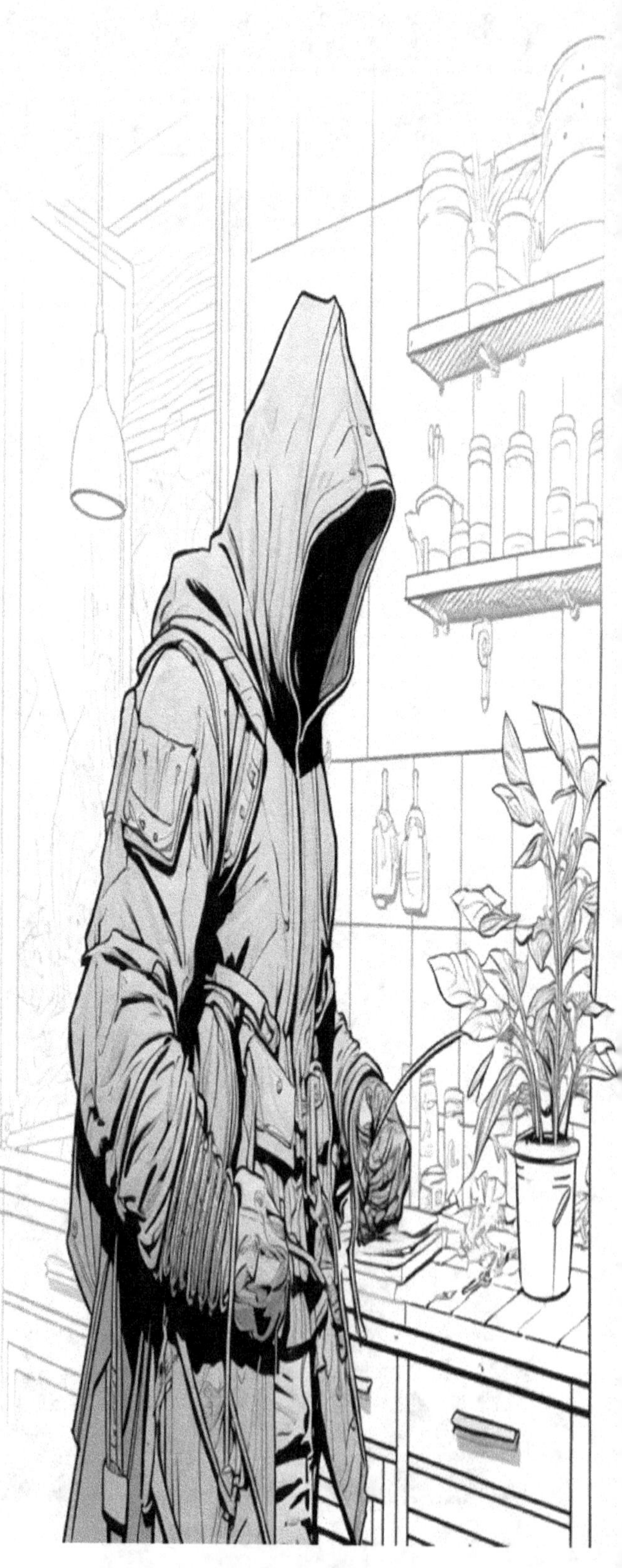

Microgreens also require less water and fertilizer than traditional gardening, making them a sustainable and eco-friendly option.

Finally, growing microgreens is a fun and rewarding hobby that can provide you with fresh, nutritious greens year-round. It's a great way to connect with nature and to experience the satisfaction of growing your own food.

In the next chapter, we will discuss how to choose the right containers for your microgreen garden, including size, material, and drainage.

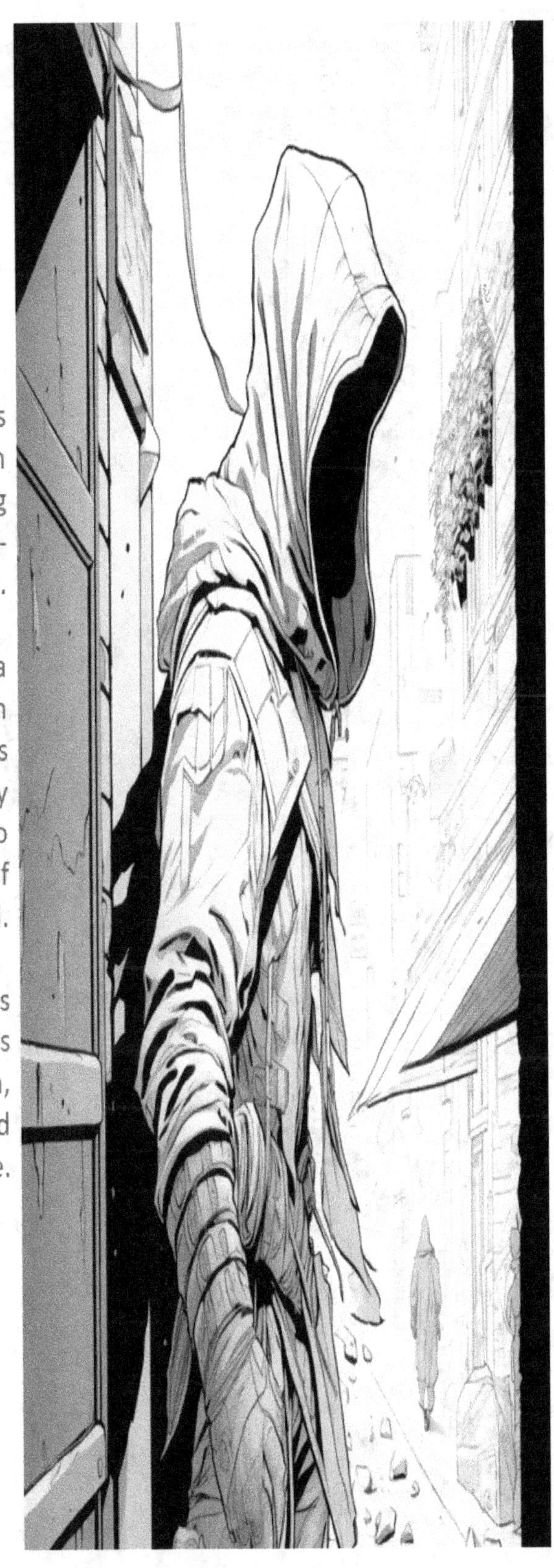

CHAPTER 3: CHOOSING THE RIGHT CONTAINERS FOR YOUR MICROGREEN GARDEN

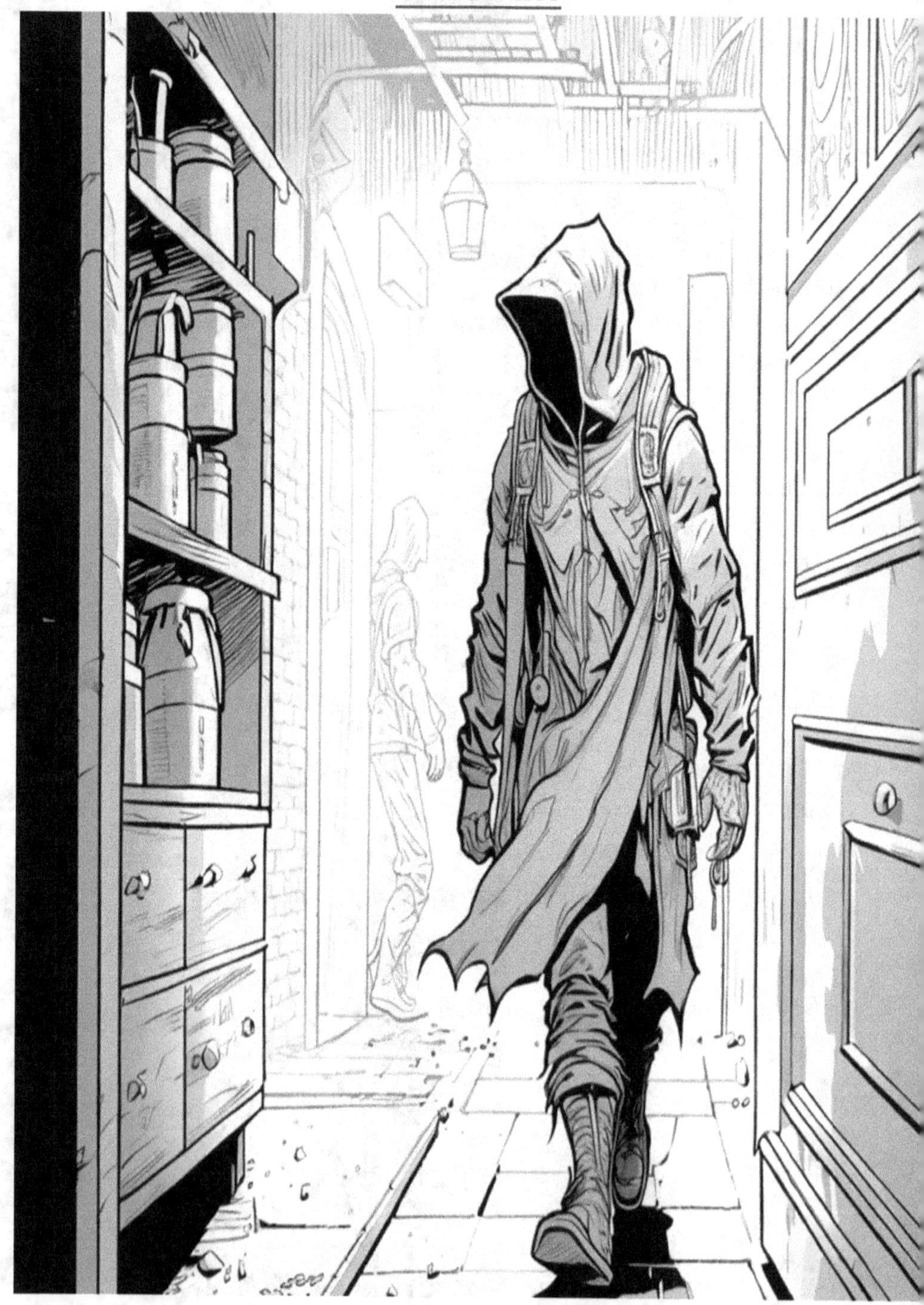

When it comes to growing microgreens, choosing the right container is important. You want a container that is the right size for your needs, made from a suitable material, and has good drainage to prevent waterlogging

Size: The size of your container will depend on the number of microgreens you want to grow and the space you have available. For small-scale indoor gardening, trays or containers that are 10-20 inches long and 4-6 inches wide are ideal. For outdoor gardening or larger-scale indoor gardening, you may want to consider larger containers or even raised beds

Material: The material of your container can impact the growth and health of your microgreens. Plastic containers are lightweight, durable, and easy to clean, but they may not be as breathable as other materials. Ceramic and clay containers are porous and can allow for better air circulation, but they may break more easily. Wooden containers are a good option for those who want a natural look, but they may not last as long as other materials

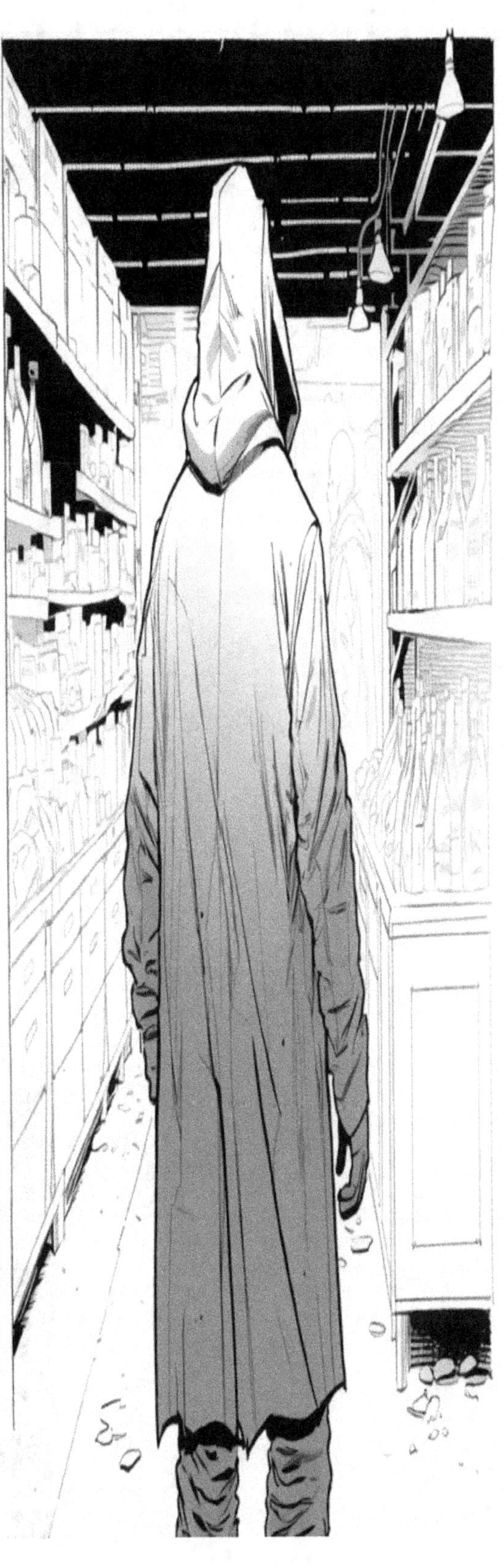

<u>**Drainage:**</u> Good drainage is crucial for the health of your microgreens. You want to make sure that excess water can drain out of the container so that the roots don't become waterlogged. To ensure good drainage, choose a container with drainage holes at the bottom or create your own drainage holes by drilling or punching holes in the bottom.

In addition to these factors, you may also want to consider the aesthetic appeal of your container. Choose a container that matches your décor or adds a pop of color to your space. In the next chapter, we will discuss how to select the right microgreen seeds for your garden, including how to choose the best seeds and how to store them.

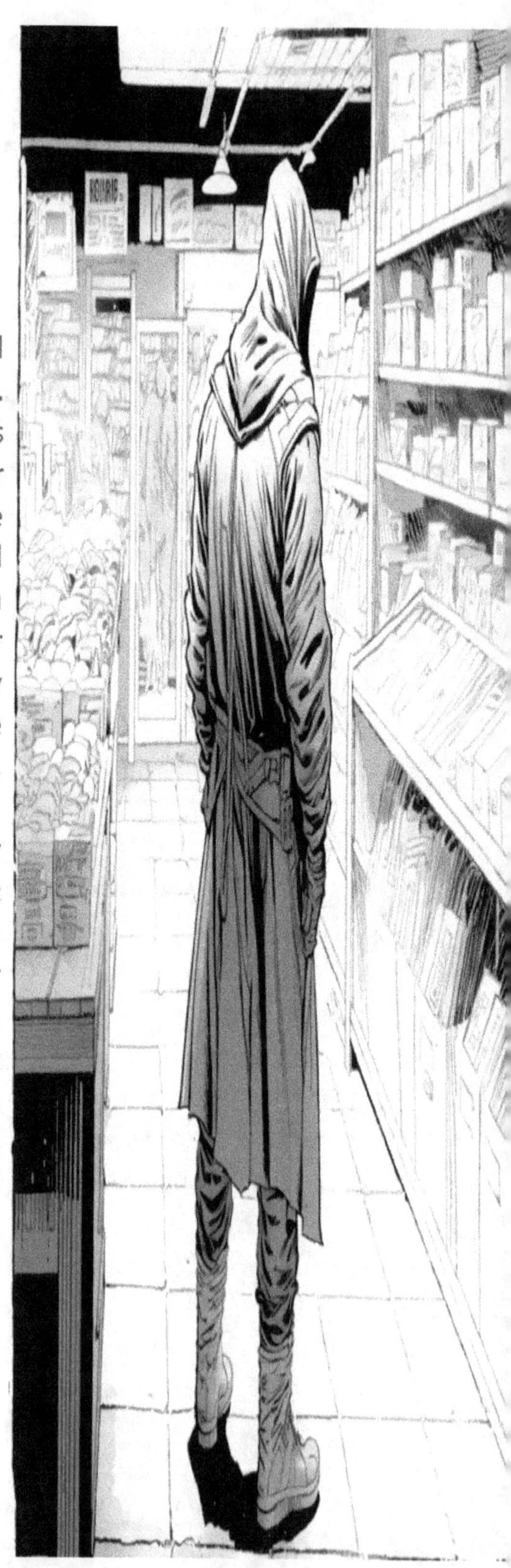

CHAPTER 4: SELECTING THE RIGHT MICROGREEN SEEDS

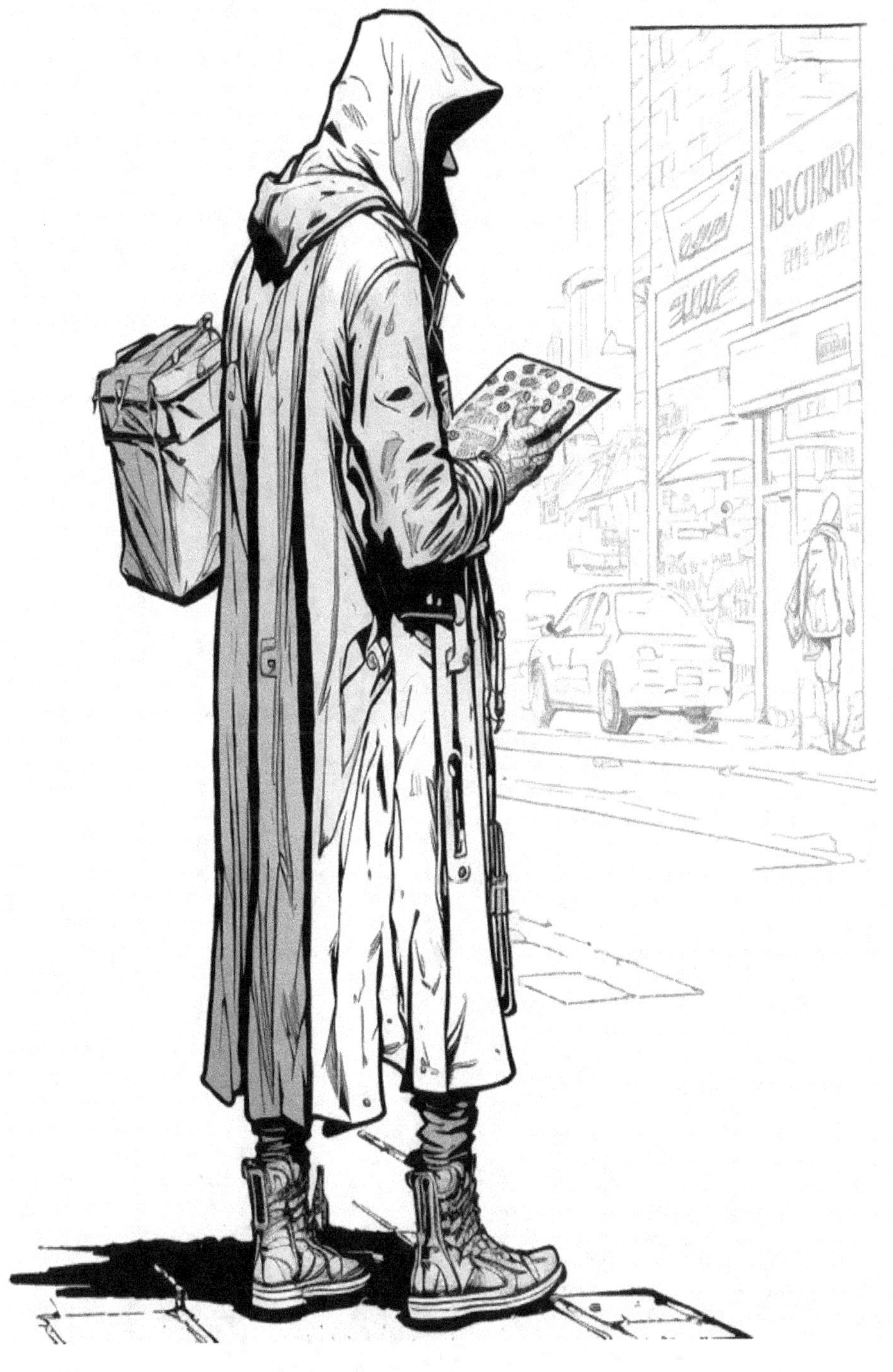

Choosing the right seeds is an important step in growing healthy and flavorful microgreens. Here are some tips for selecting the best seeds for your microgreen garden.

Choose high-quality seeds: Look for seeds that are fresh and of high quality. Seeds that are past their expiration date or have been stored improperly may not germinate as well or produce healthy plants.

Choose the right variety: There are many different types of microgreens to choose from, each with their own unique flavor and nutritional profile. Consider what types of microgreens you enjoy and what you plan to use them for when selecting your seeds.

Choose organic seeds: Organic seeds are grown without the use of harmful chemicals or pesticides, making them a healthier choice for you and the environment.

Store your seeds properly: To ensure that your seeds remain viable, store them in a cool, dry place, away from direct sunlight. Airtight containers or zip-top bags can help to protect your seeds from moisture and pests. In addition to these tips, you may also want to consider purchasing seed kits that include everything you need to

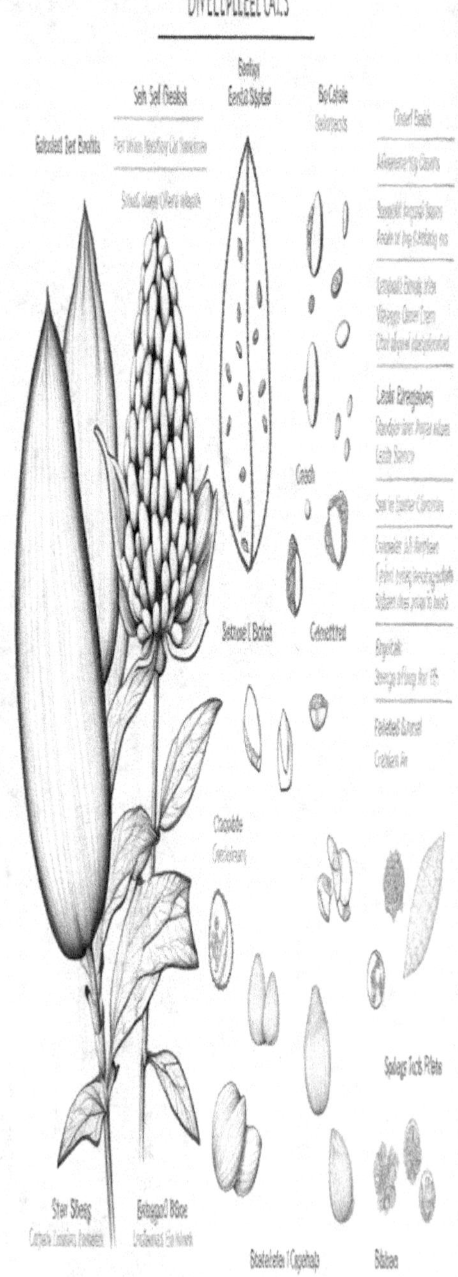

start growing your microgreens, including seeds, growing medium, and instructions. Seed kits are a great option for beginners who are new to microgreen gardening.
In the next chapter, we will discuss how to prepare your soil or growing medium for your microgreen garden.

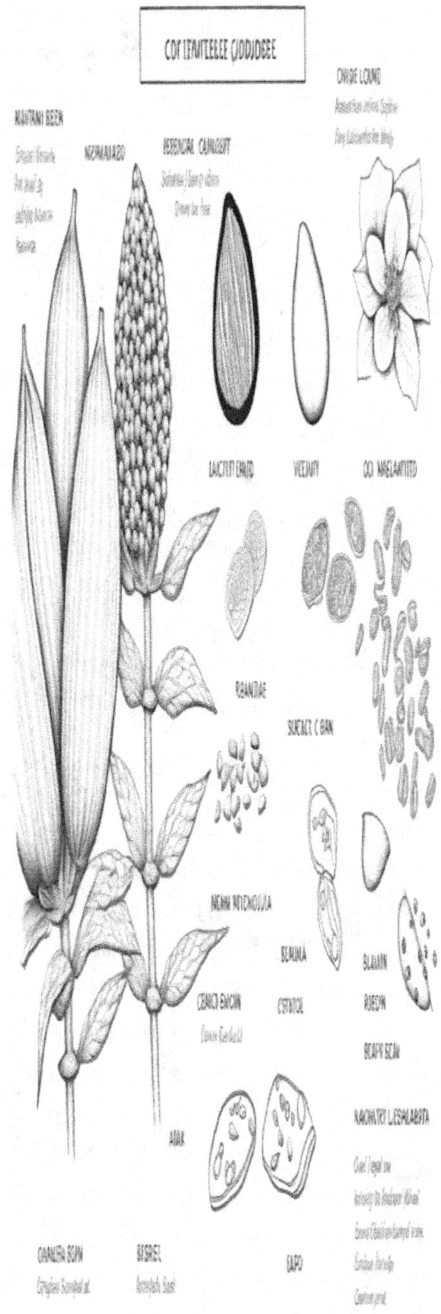

CHAPTER 5: SOIL AND GROWING MEDIUM FOR MICROGREENS

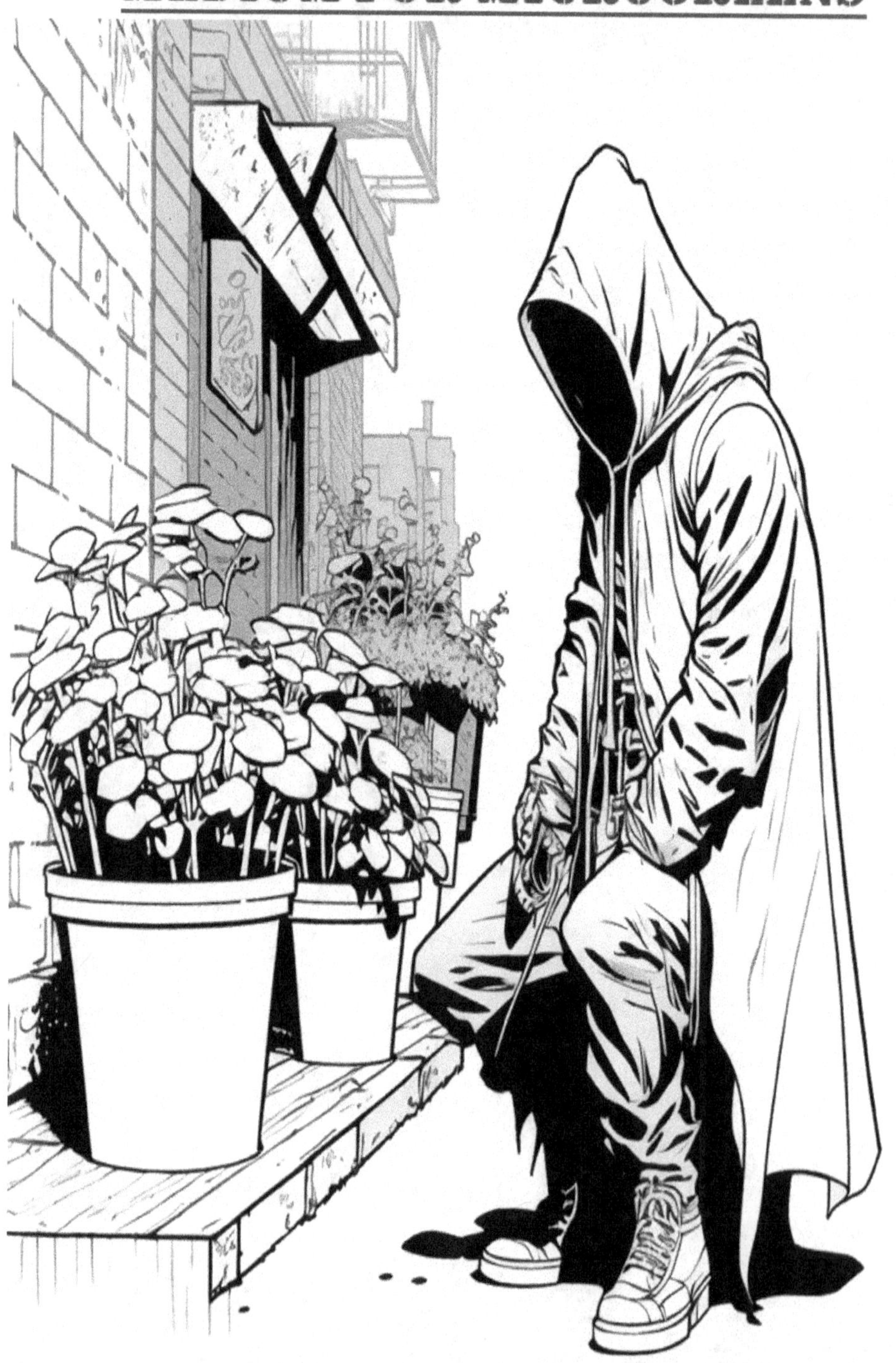

When it comes to growing microgreens, the right soil or growing medium is crucial for the health and growth of your plants. Here are some tips for selecting and preparing your soil or growing medium:

Select a suitable growing medium: While soil is a common growing medium for traditional gardening, it may not be the best choice for microgreens. Instead, consider using a soilless growing medium, such as coconut coir, peat moss, or vermiculite. These materials are lightweight, absorbent, and provide good aeration for your plants.

Prepare your growing medium: If you are using a soilless growing medium, you will need to prepare it before planting your seeds. Follow the instructions on the package to hydrate the medium and fluff it up. You may also want to add some organic fertilizer or compost to provide nutrients for your plants.

Fill your containers: Once your growing medium is prepared, fill your containers with a layer

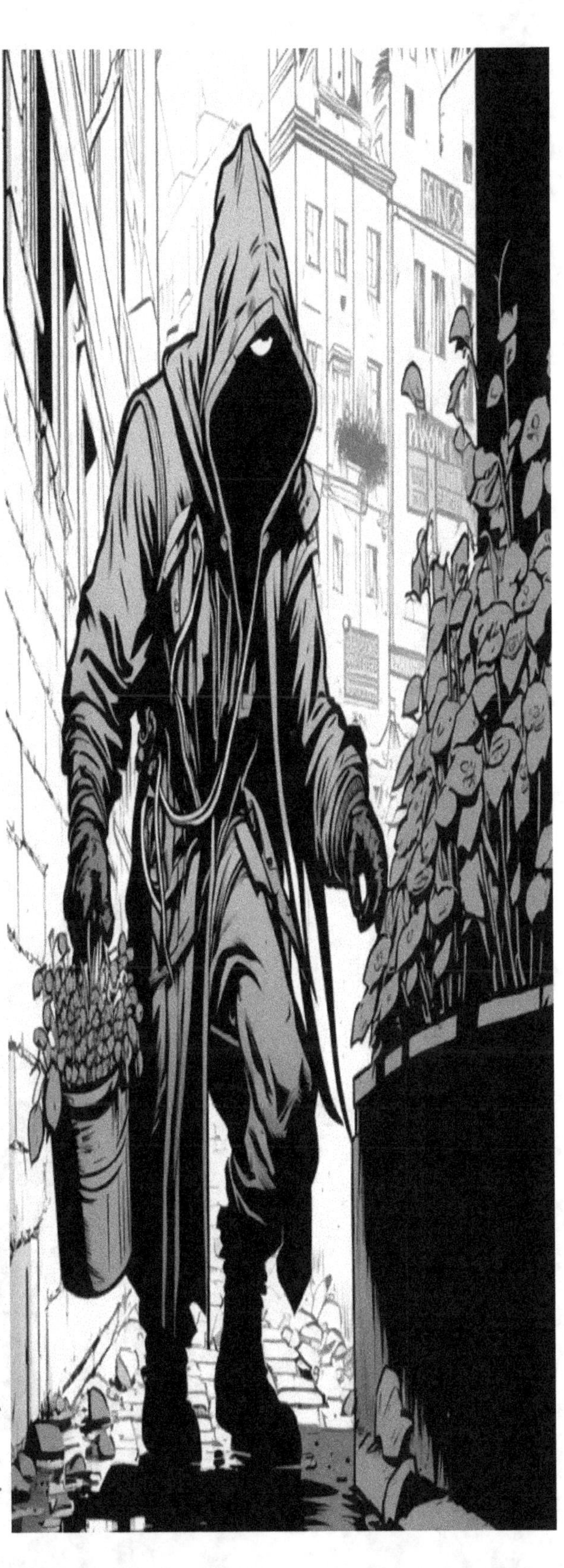

Of about 1-2 inches of the medium.
Make sure to leave enough space at
the top for your seeds to germinate
and grow.

In addition to these tips, you may also
want to consider adding a drainage
layer to the bottom of your container
to help prevent waterlogging. This
can be done by adding a layer of
gravel or sand to the bottom of the
container before adding your growing
medium.

In the next chapter, we will discuss
how to water your microgreens and
how to ensure that they get the right
amount of moisture for optimal
growth.

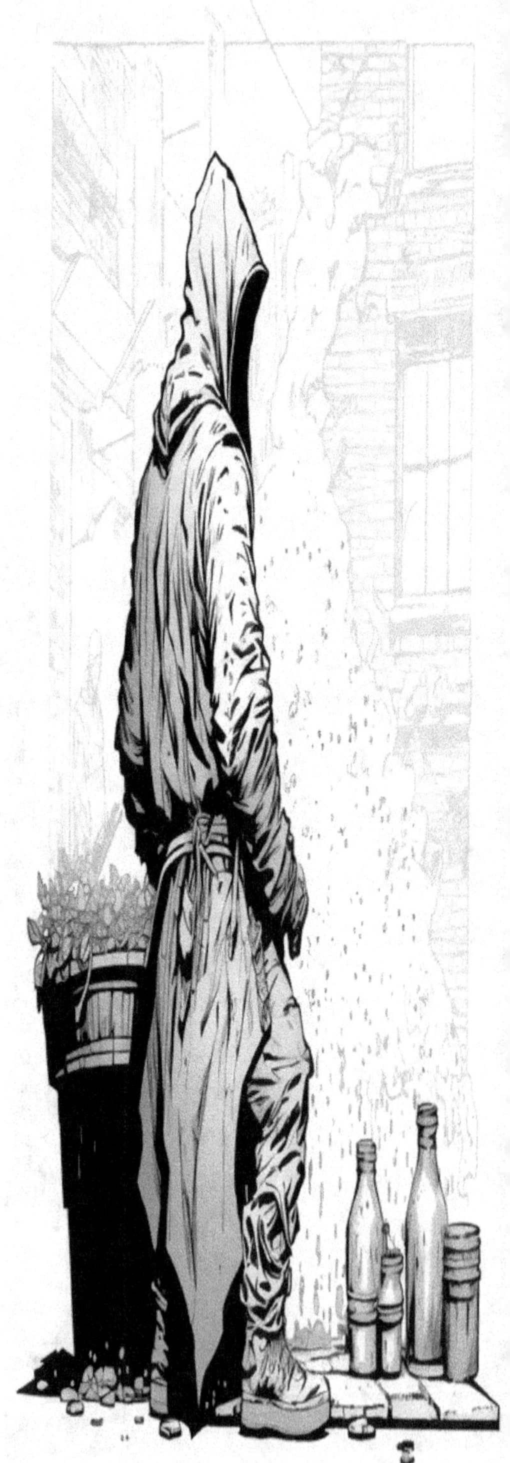

CHAPTER 6: WATERING YOUR MICROGREENS

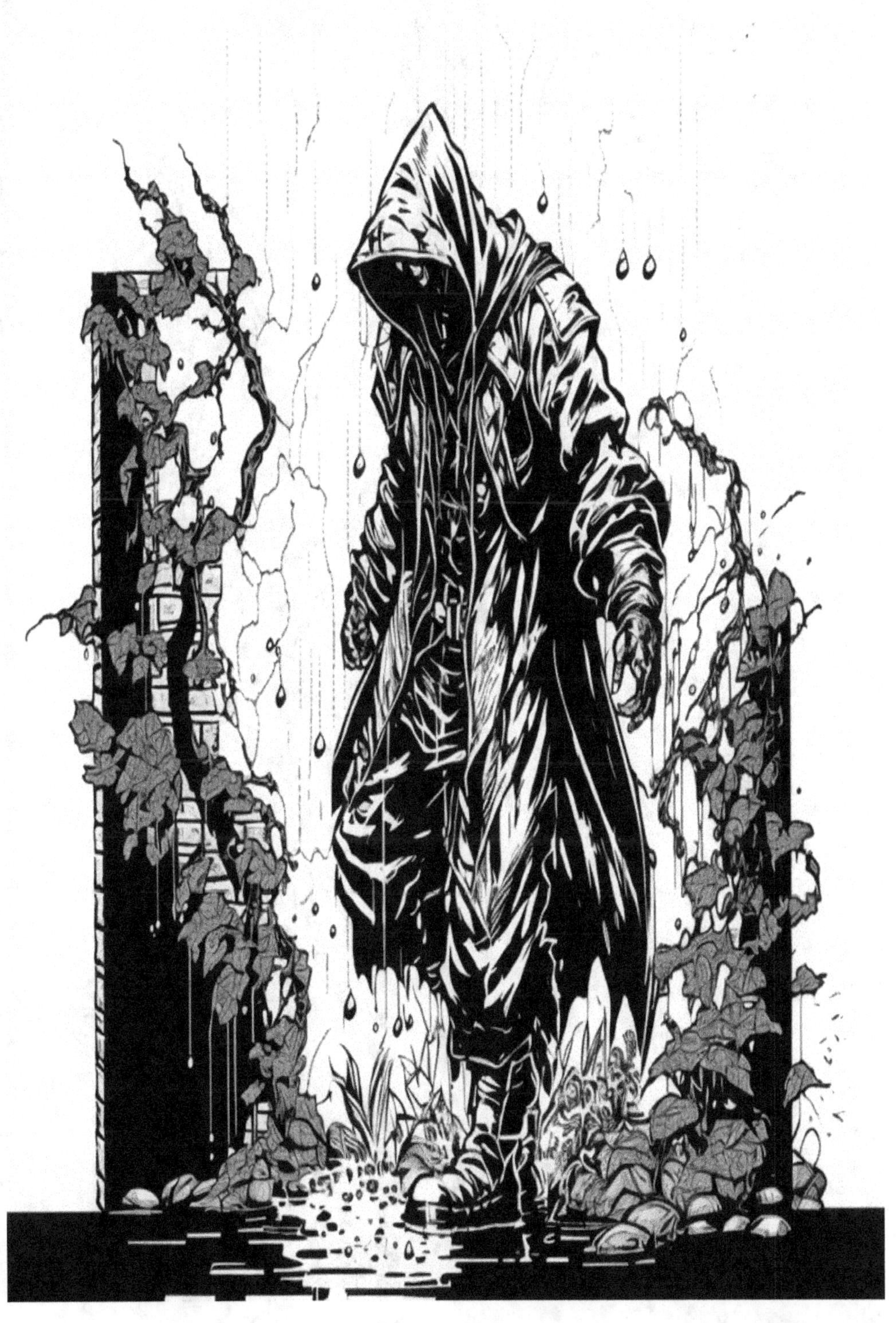

Proper watering is crucial for the health and growth of your microgreens. Here are some tips for watering your microgreens:

Water your microgreens from the bottom: Instead of watering from the top, which can disturb the soil or growing medium and may cause damage to your microgreens, water your microgreens from the bottom. This can be done by placing your container in a tray or dish filled with water and allowing the water to soak up through the drainage holes.

Don't overwater: Overwatering can lead to waterlogging, which can cause root rot and other problems. Make sure to check the moisture level of your soil or growing medium regularly and only water when it feels dry to the touch.

Provide adequate drainage: make sure that your container has good drainage. This can be done by ensuring that there are enough drainage holes at the bottom of your micro container and by adding a layer of gravel or sand to the bottom of the drainage container.

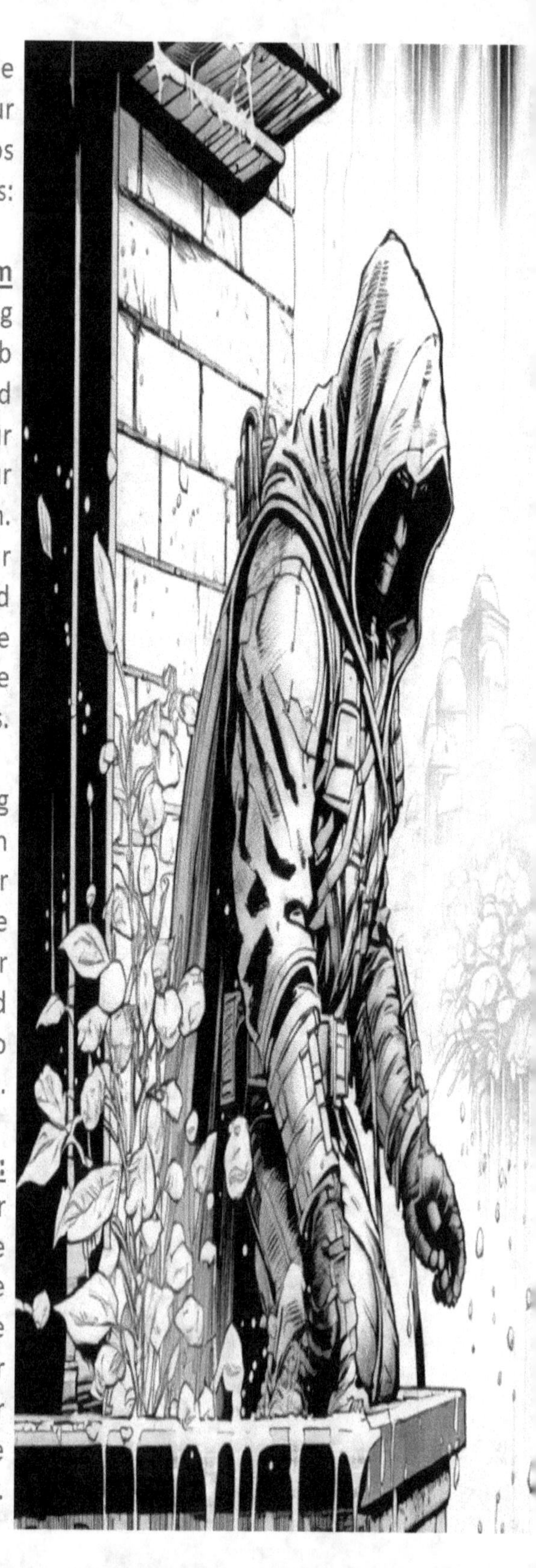

<u>**Use filtered or distilled water**</u>: Tap water can contain chlorine or other chemicals that can be harmful to your microgreens. Consider using filtered or distilled water instead to ensure that your microgreens get the purest water possible.

In addition to these tips, you may also want to consider using a spray bottle or misting your microgreens with water to provide additional moisture. This can be especially helpful during the germination phase when the seeds are just starting to sprout.

In the next chapter, we will discuss lighting for your microgreen garden, including the amount of light that microgreens need and how to provide the right type of light for optimal growth.

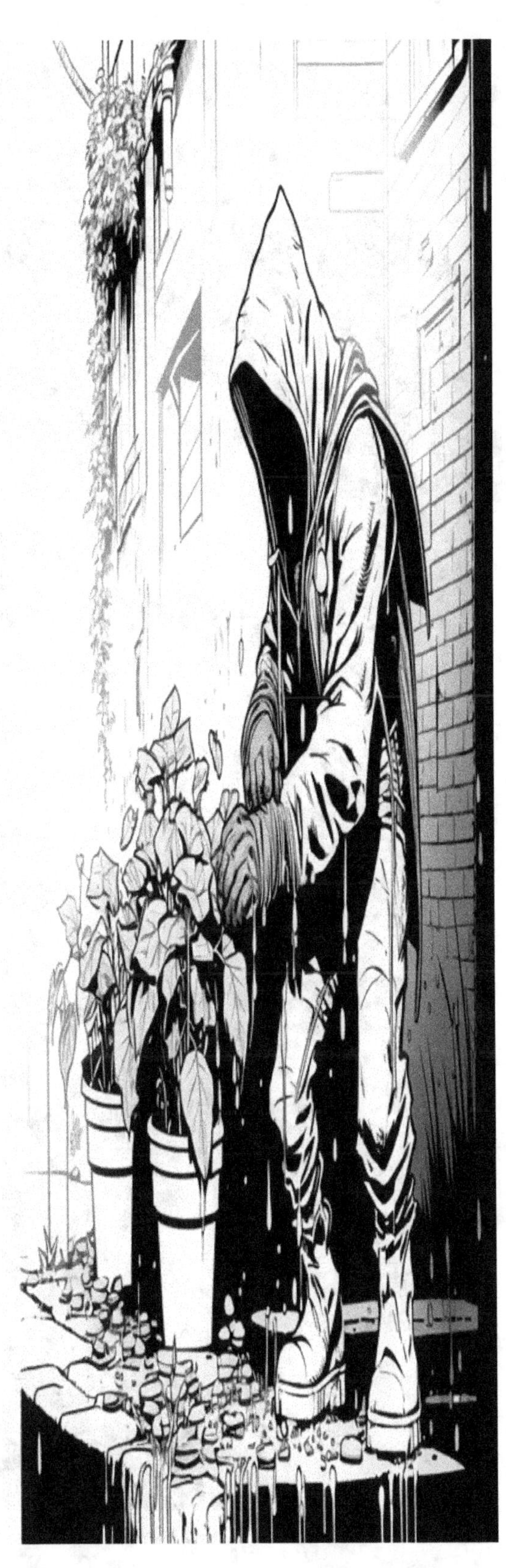

CHAPTER 7: LIGHTING FOR YOUR MICROGREEN GARDEN

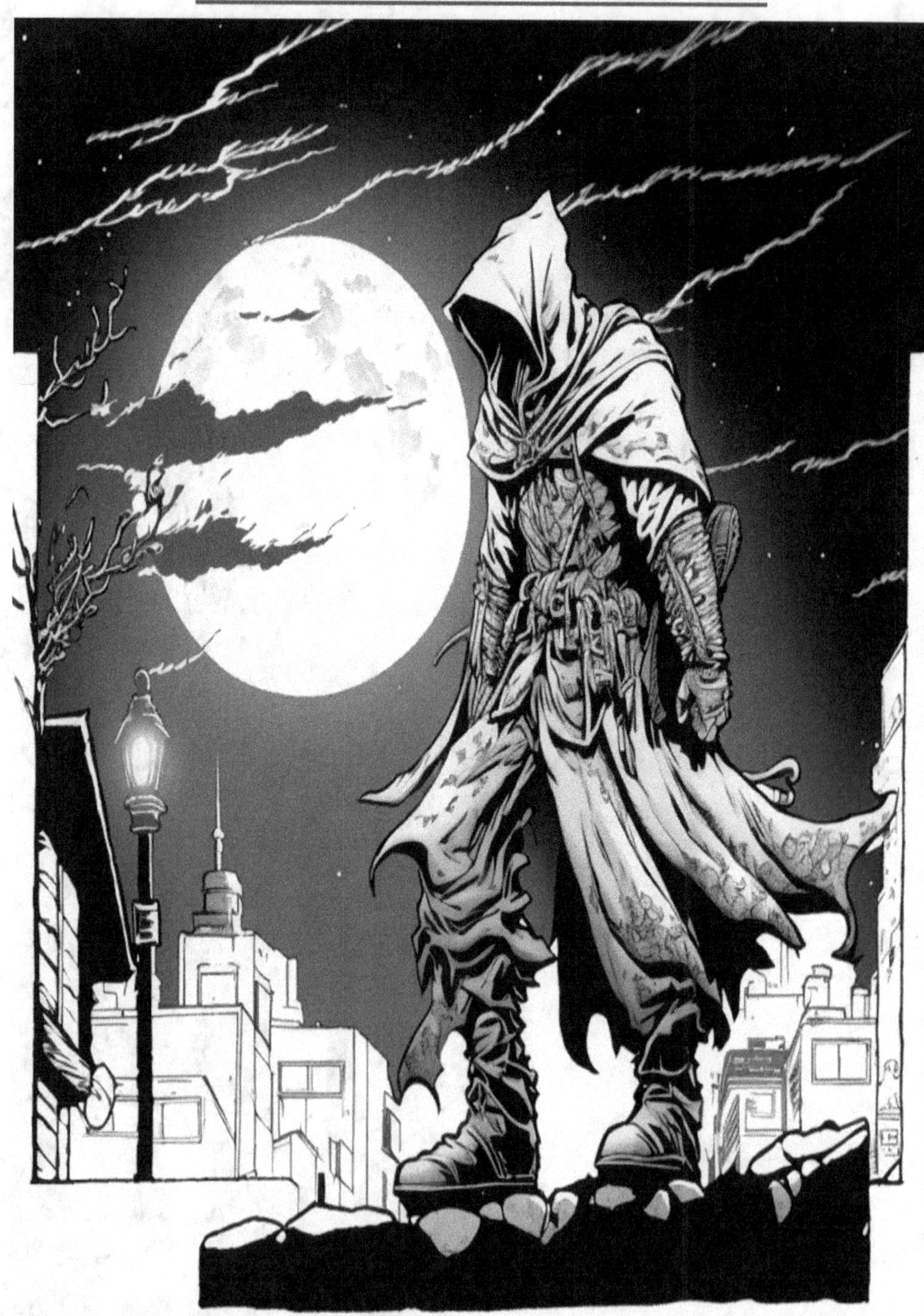

Lighting is an essential factor in the growth and development of your microgreens. Here are some tips for providing the right amount and type of light for your microgreen garden:

Amount of light: Microgreens need a lot of light to grow properly. Ideally, they should receive 12-16 hours of light each day. If you are growing your microgreens indoors, you may need to use artificial light sources to provide enough light.

Type of light: Microgreens can grow under a variety of light sources, including natural light, fluorescent lights, or LED lights. Natural light is the most ideal, but if you are growing your microgreens indoors, you may need to use artificial light

sources to provide enough light. Fluorescent lights and LED lights are both good options for indoor growing, as they are energy-efficient and provide a good spectrum of light for plant growth.

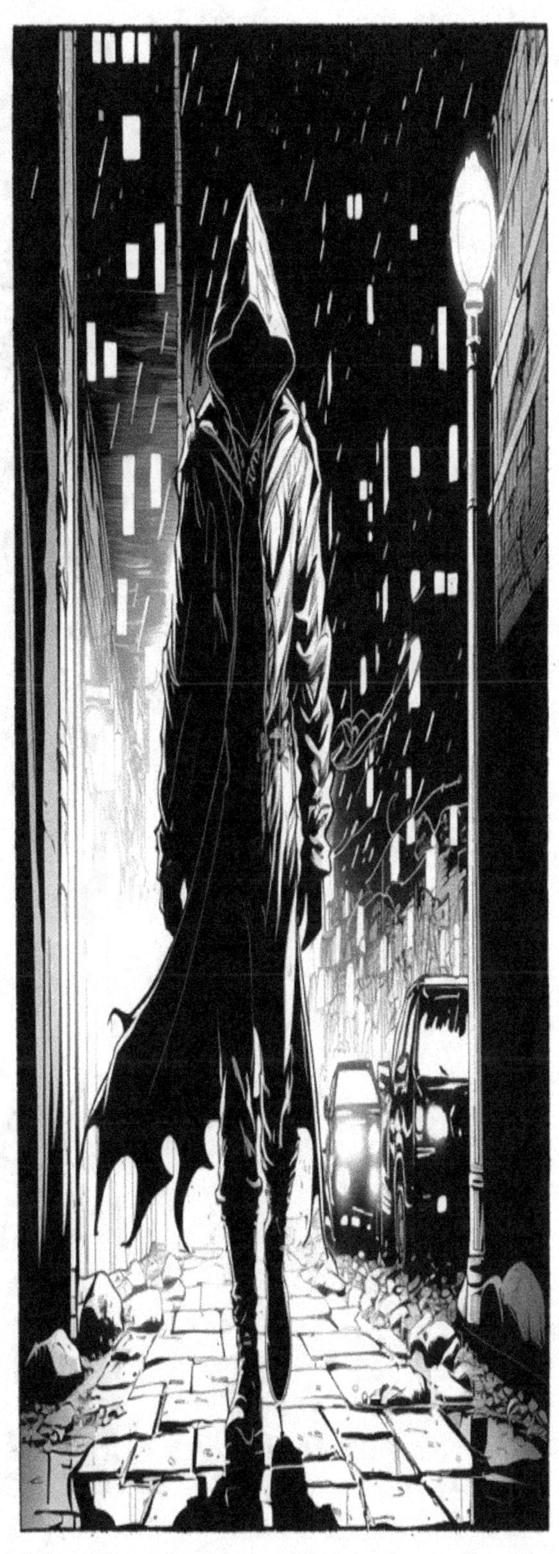

<u>**Distance from light source:**</u> The distance between your microgreens and the light source is also important. If the light source is too far away, your microgreens may not receive enough light. If the light source is too close, your microgreens may become overheated and burn. Aim to keep your light source 2-4 inches away from your microgreens.

<u>**Lighting schedule:**</u> It's important to provide consistent lighting for your microgreens. If you are using artificial lighting, you may want to use a timer to ensure that your microgreens receive the proper amount of light each day.

In addition to these tips, you may also want to consider rotating your microgreens regularly to ensure that all parts of the plant receive adequate light. This can be done by turning your container a quarter-turn every day or two.

In the next chapter, we will discuss how to plant your microgreens, including how to sow your seeds, cover them, and germinate them.

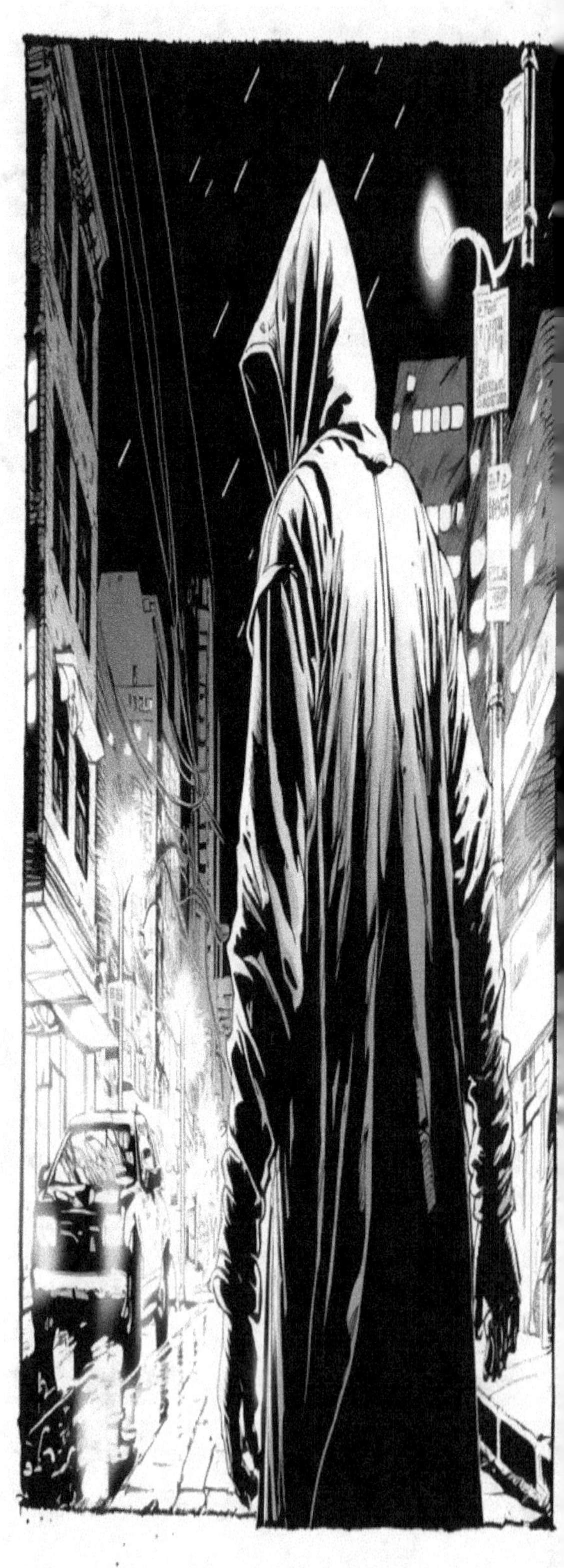

CHAPTER 8: PLANTING YOUR MICROGREENS

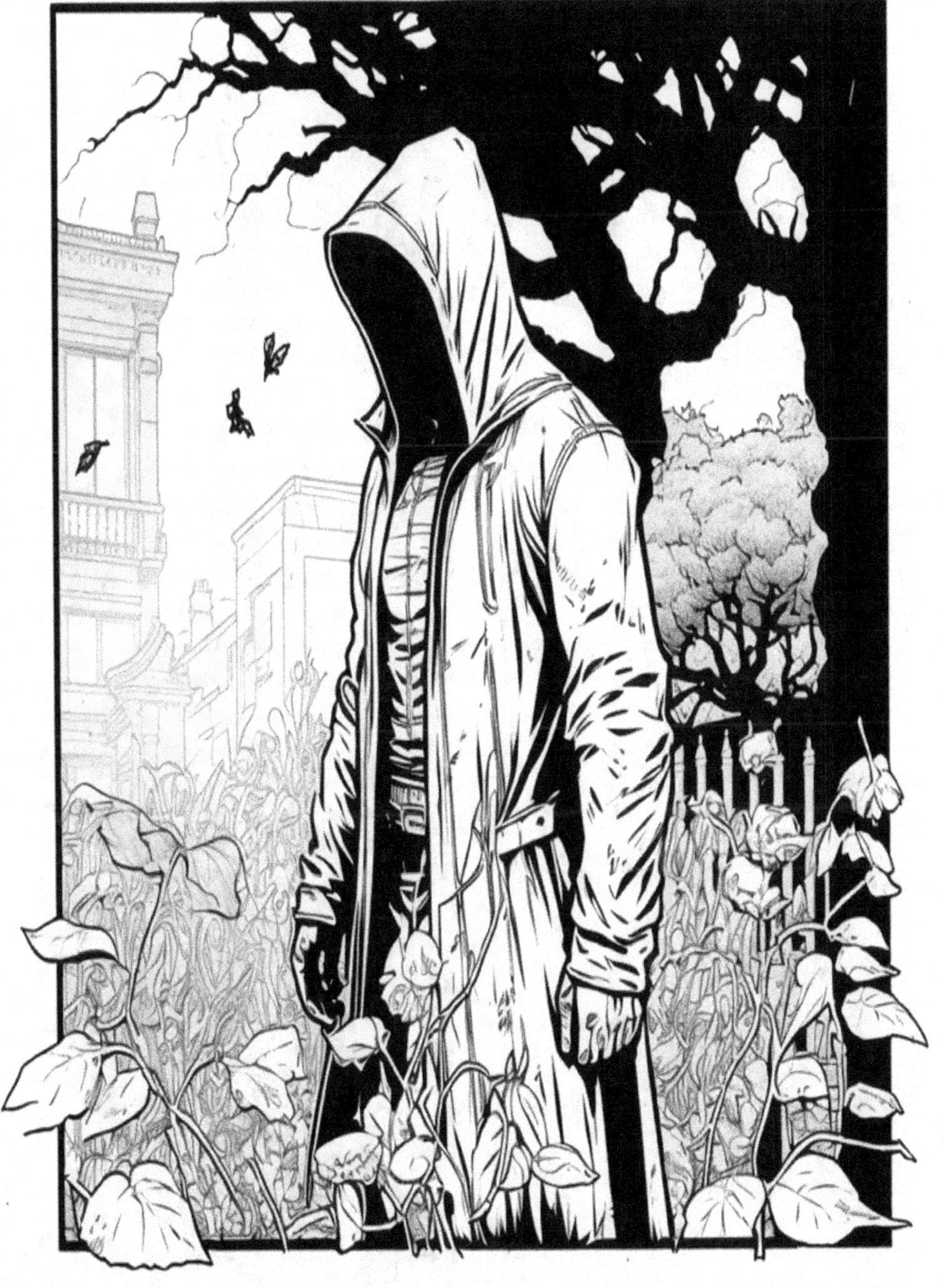

Planting your microgreens is a simple process that can be done in just a few easy steps. Here's how to plant your microgreens:

1.<u>Sow your seeds:</u> Sprinkle your seeds evenly over the surface of your growing medium, making sure to leave some space between each seed. Depending on the variety of microgreens, you may need to adjust the density of the seeds.

2.<u>Cover your seeds:</u> Cover your seeds with a thin layer of growing medium to protect them from drying out and to provide some insulation for the germination process. Use a spray bottle to mist the top layer of soil to settle it around the seeds.

3.<u>Germinate your seeds:</u> Place your container in a warm, well-lit area, and keep the soil moist but not too wet. Germination should occur within a few days to a week, depending on the variety of microgreens.

4.<u>Uncover your seeds:</u> Once your seeds have germinated and have grown to about 1-2 inches in height, remove the covering layer of soil to allow the microgreens to receive light and air.

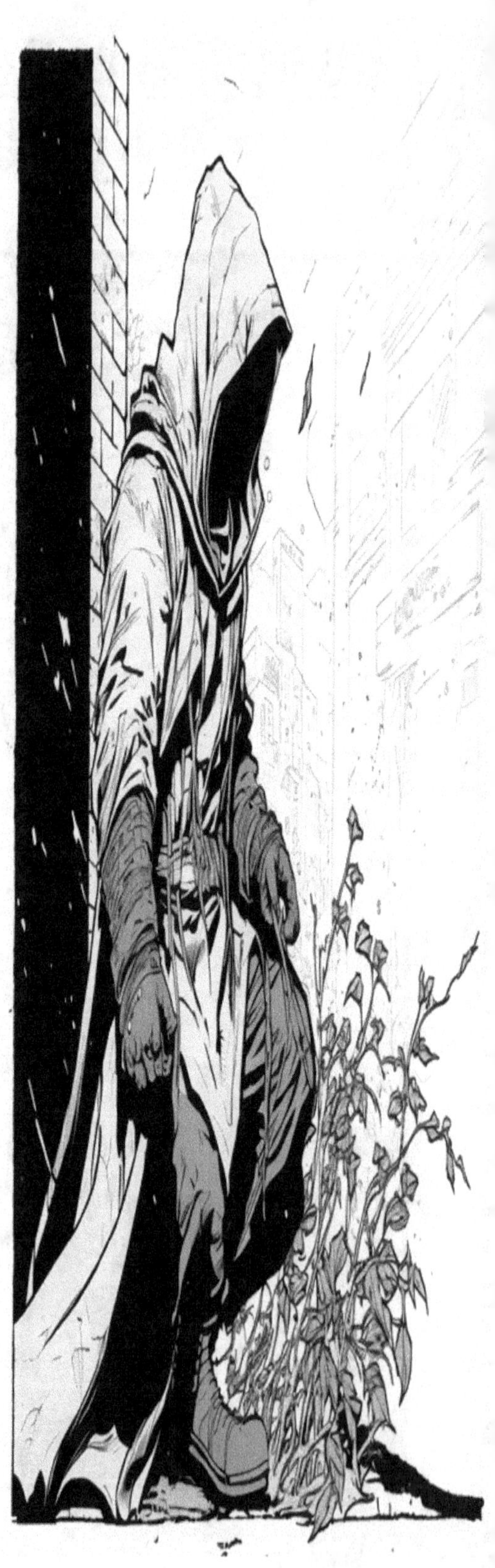

5.Water and fertilize as needed:
Water your microgreens from the bottom as needed, making sure not to overwater. You may also want to fertilize your microgreens with a dilute solution of organic fertilizer or compost tea.

6.Harvest your microgreens:
Harvest your microgreens once they have reached the desired height, usually around 1-3 inches. Use a clean pair of scissors or a sharp knife to cut the microgreens just above the soil line.

In the next chapter, we will discuss common problems that can occur when growing microgreens and how to troubleshoot them.

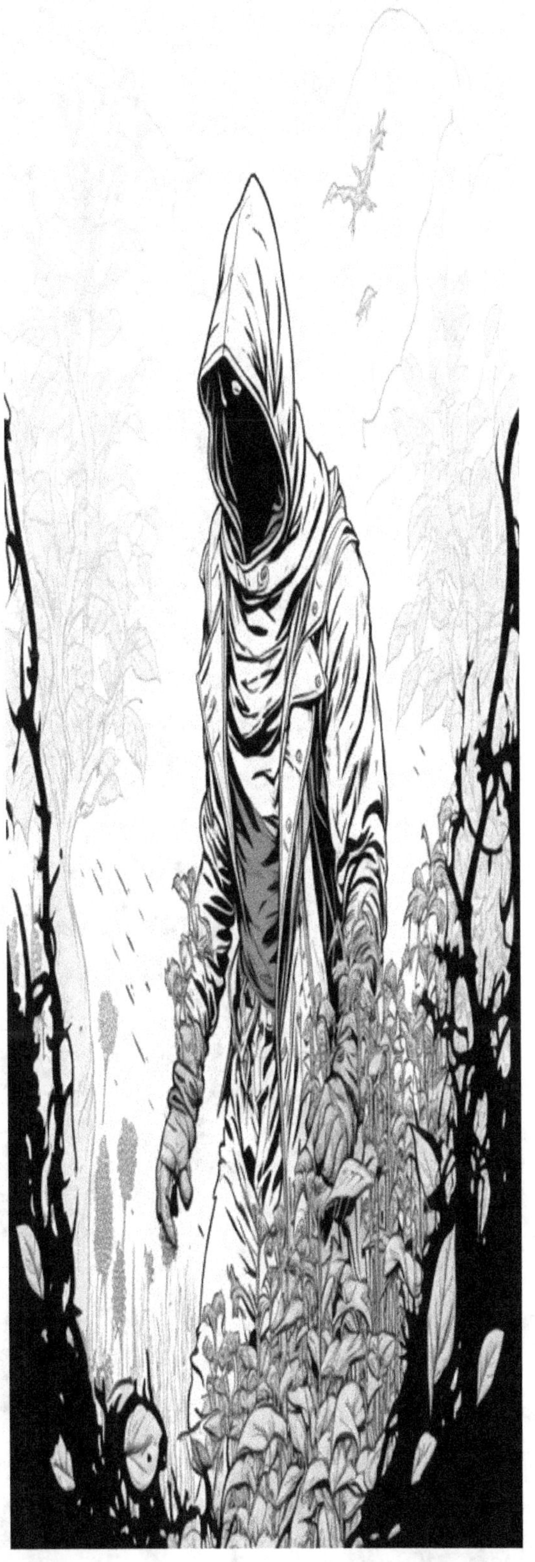

CHAPTER 9: TROUBLESHOOTING COMMON PROBLEMS WITH MICROGREENS

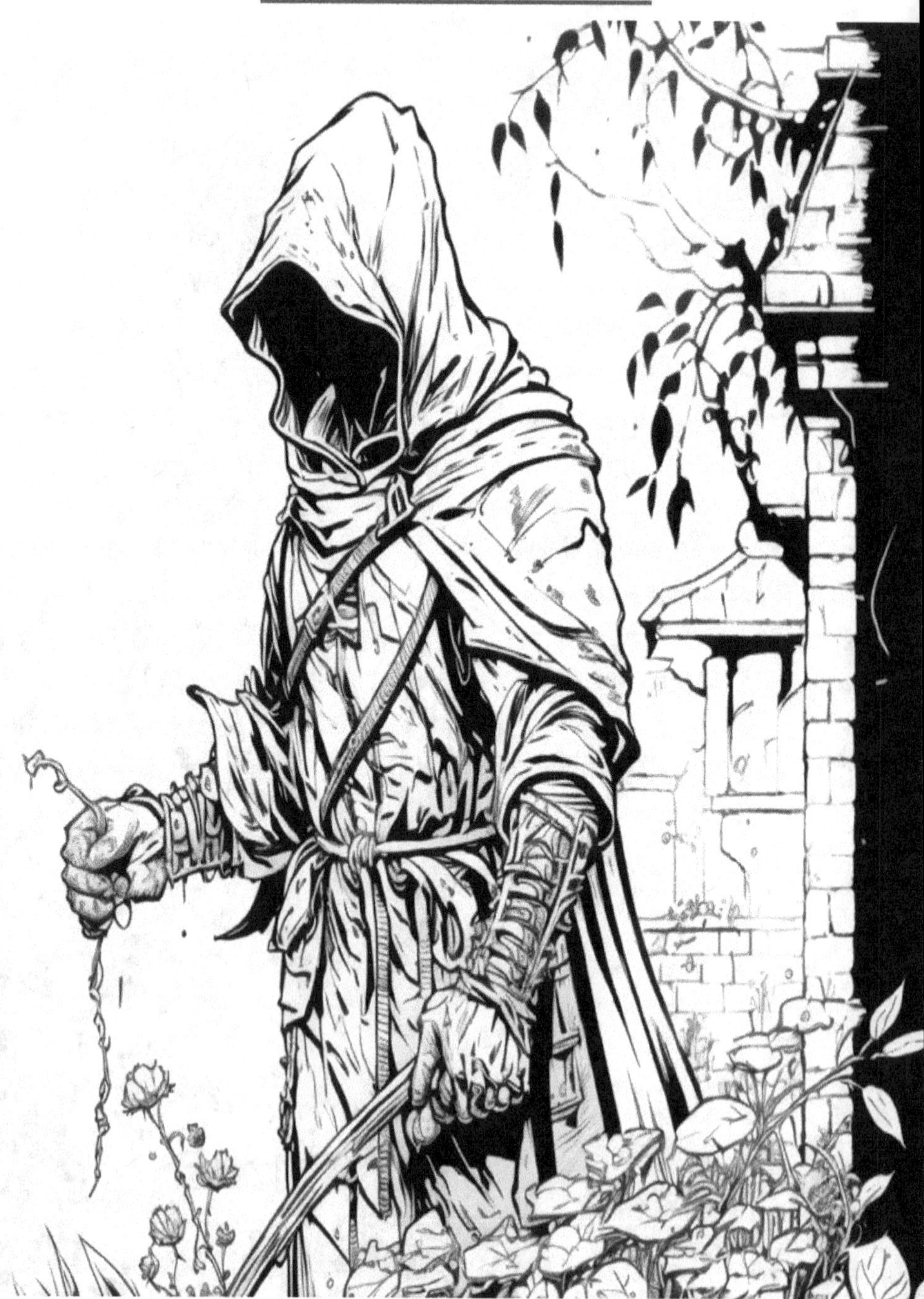

While growing microgreens is generally easy and straightforward, there are some common problems that you may encounter. Here are some tips for troubleshooting these problems:

Problem: Slow germination. **Solution:** Make sure that your seeds are fresh and of high quality, and that your growing medium is moist but not too wet. You may also want to try soaking your seeds in water for a few hours before planting to help speed up germination.

Problem: Yellowing or wilting of leaves. Solution: This can be a sign of overwatering or underwatering. Make sure to check the moisture level of your soil or growing medium regularly and adjust your watering accordingly. Yellowing leaves can also be a sign of nutrient deficiency, so you may want to fertilize your microgreens with a dilute solution of organic fertilizer.

Problem: Mold or fungal growth. **Solution:** Mold or fungal growth can occur if your microgreens are too wet or if the growing environment is too humid.

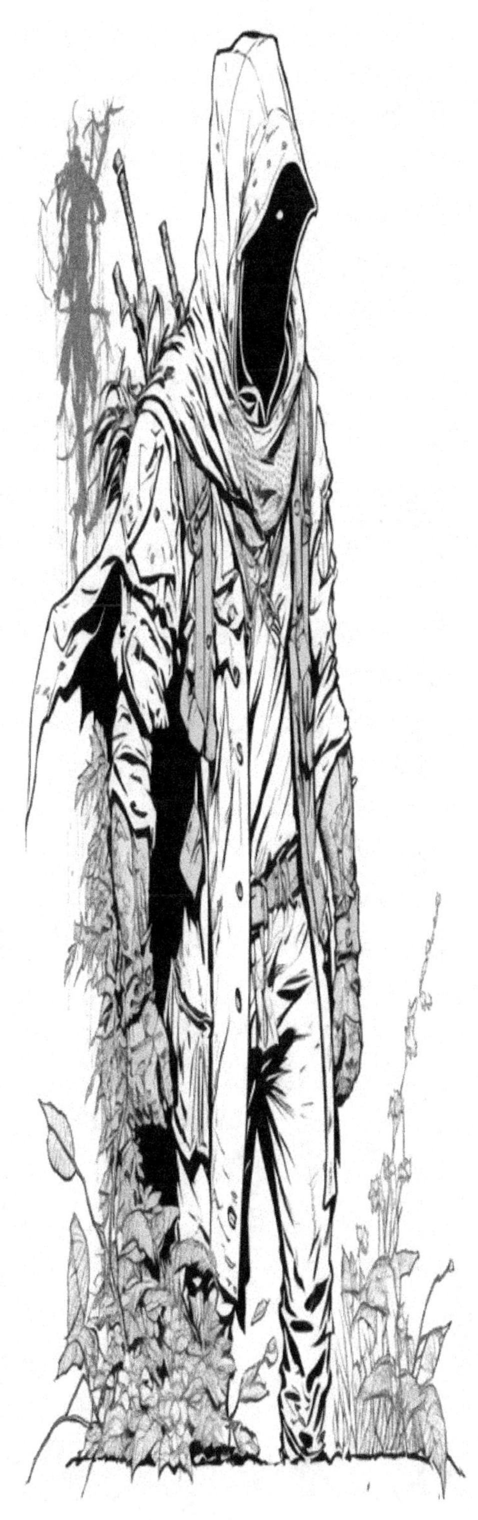

Make sure to provide adequate ventilation and air circulation and avoid overwatering your microgreens. You can also try adding a small amount of cinnamon powder to your growing medium to help prevent mold and fungal growth.

Problem: Pests such as aphids or spider mites. Solution: Pests can be a common problem with microgreens, especially if you are growing them indoors. You can try using natural pest control methods such as insecticidal soap or neem oil. Alternatively, you can cover your microgreens with a mesh or netting to prevent pests from accessing them. By following these tips, you can help ensure that your microgreens stay healthy and vibrant. In the next chapter, we will discuss different varieties of microgreens and their unique flavors and nutritional profiles.

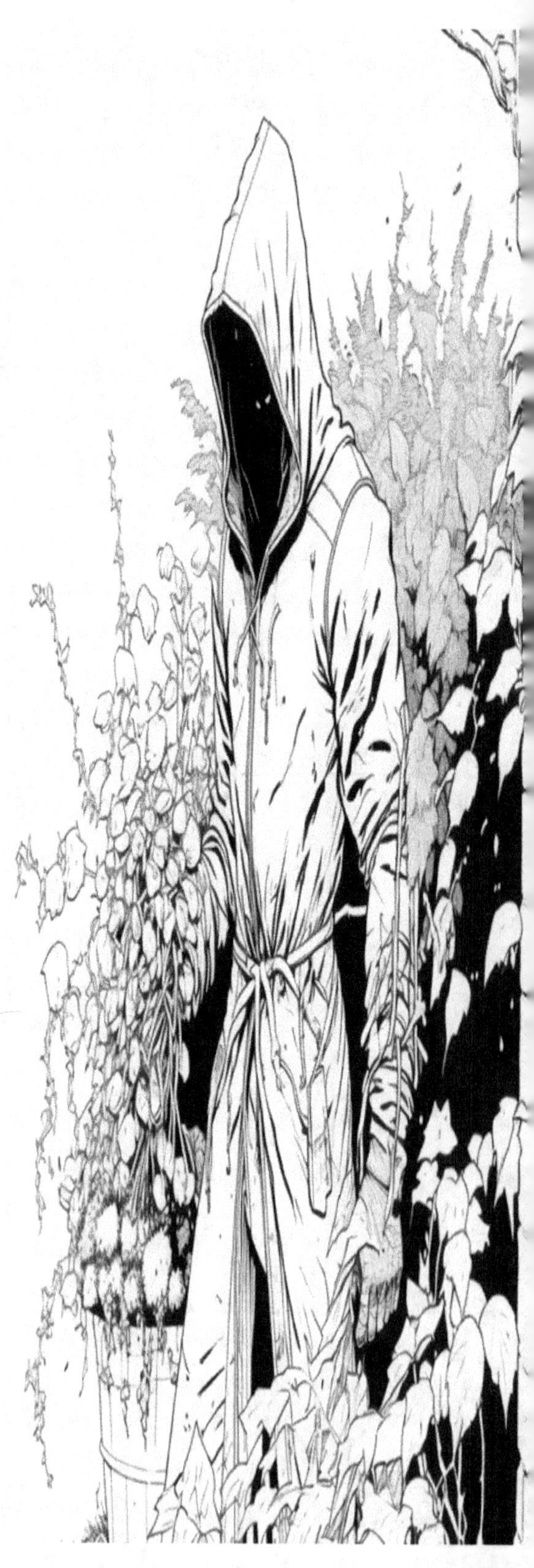

CHAPTER 10: VARIETIES OF MICROGREENS

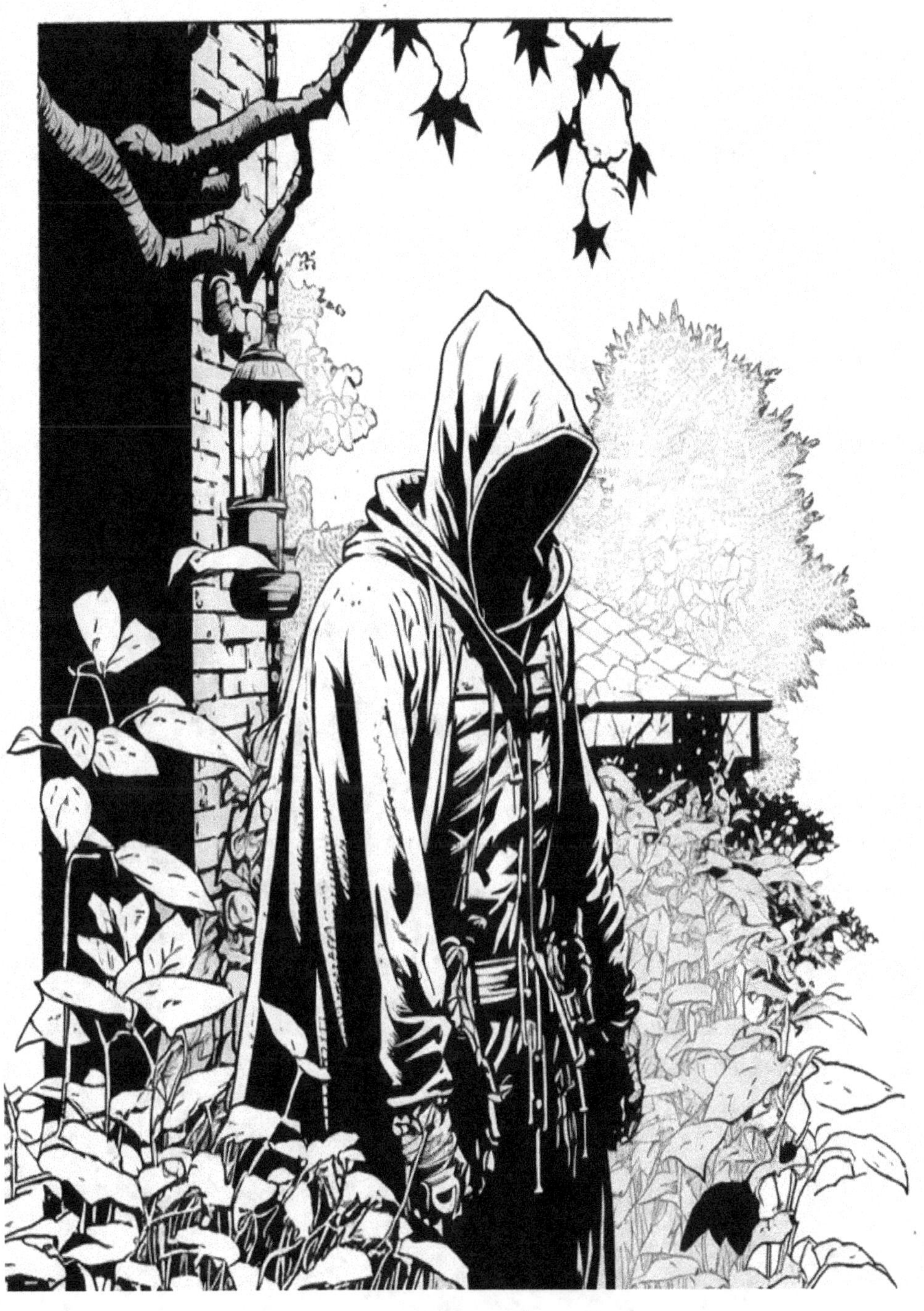

There are many different varieties of microgreens to choose from, each with their own unique flavors and nutritional profiles. Here are some of the most popular varieties of microgreens:

1.<u>Arugula:</u> Arugula microgreens have a spicy, peppery flavor and are a good source of vitamin C, calcium, and iron.

2.<u>Broccoli:</u> Broccoli microgreens have a mild, nutty flavor and are a good source of vitamin A, vitamin C, and calcium.

3.<u>Radish:</u> Radish microgreens have a spicy, peppery flavor and are a good source of vitamin C, potassium, and calcium.

4.<u>Sunflower:</u> Sunflower microgreens have a nutty, slightly sweet flavor and are a good source of vitamin E, magnesium, and protein.

5.<u>Wheatgrass:</u> Wheatgrass microgreens have a sweet, slightly earthy flavor and are a good source of chlorophyll, vitamin C, and antioxidants.

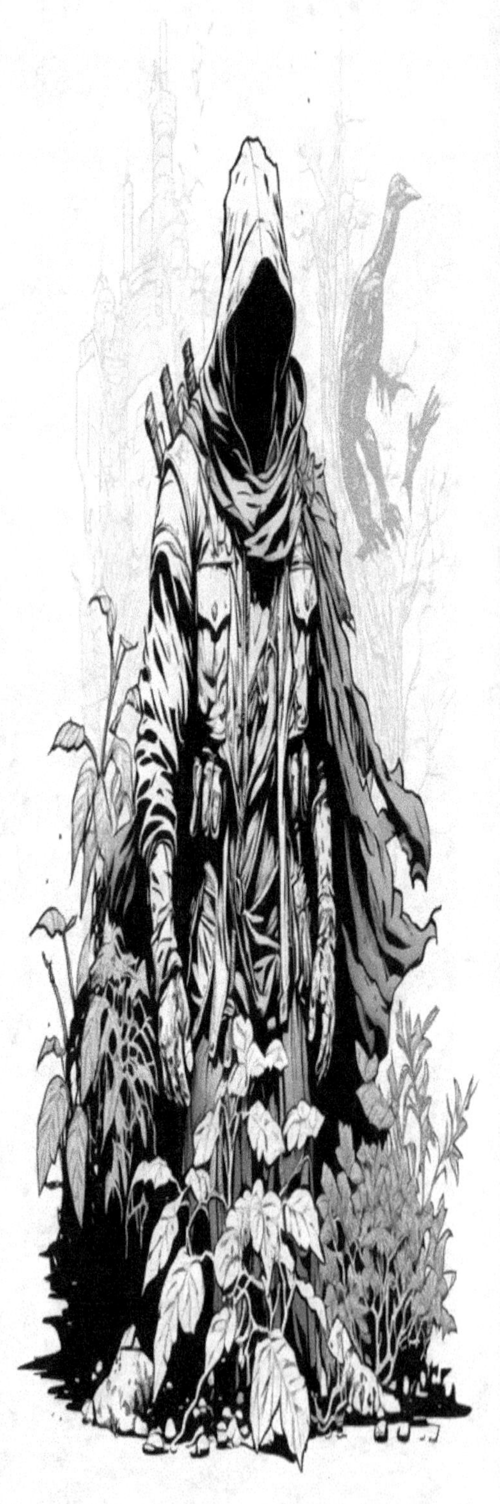

<u>**6.Beet:**</u> Beet microgreens have a slightly sweet, earthy flavor and are a good source of vitamin A, vitamin C, and iron.

<u>**7.Pea:**</u> Pea microgreens have a sweet, mild flavor and are a good source of vitamin C, vitamin K, and folate.

<u>**8.Cilantro:**</u> Cilantro microgreens have a fresh, citrusy flavor and are a good source of vitamin C, vitamin K, and antioxidants.

Experiment with different varieties of microgreens to find the flavors that you enjoy the most. You can also try mixing different varieties together to create unique flavor combinations.

In the next chapter, we will discuss the nutritional benefits of microgreens and how they can contribute to a healthy diet.

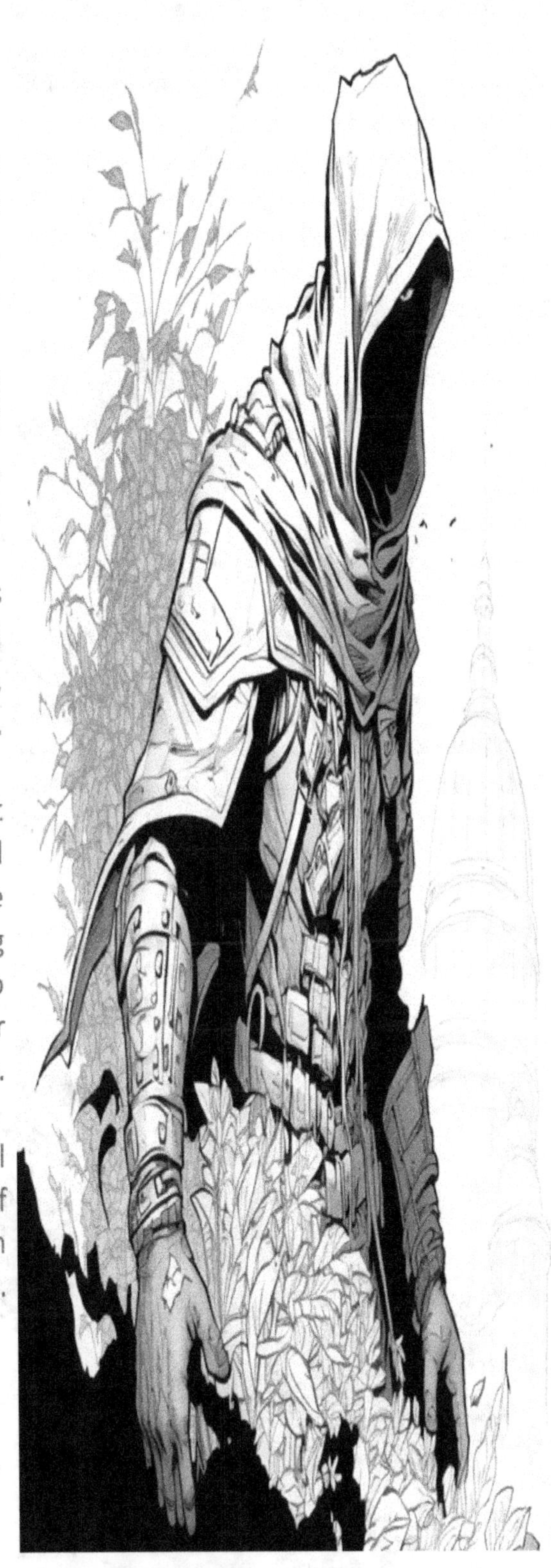

CHAPTER 11: NUTRITIONAL BENEFITS OF MICROGREENS

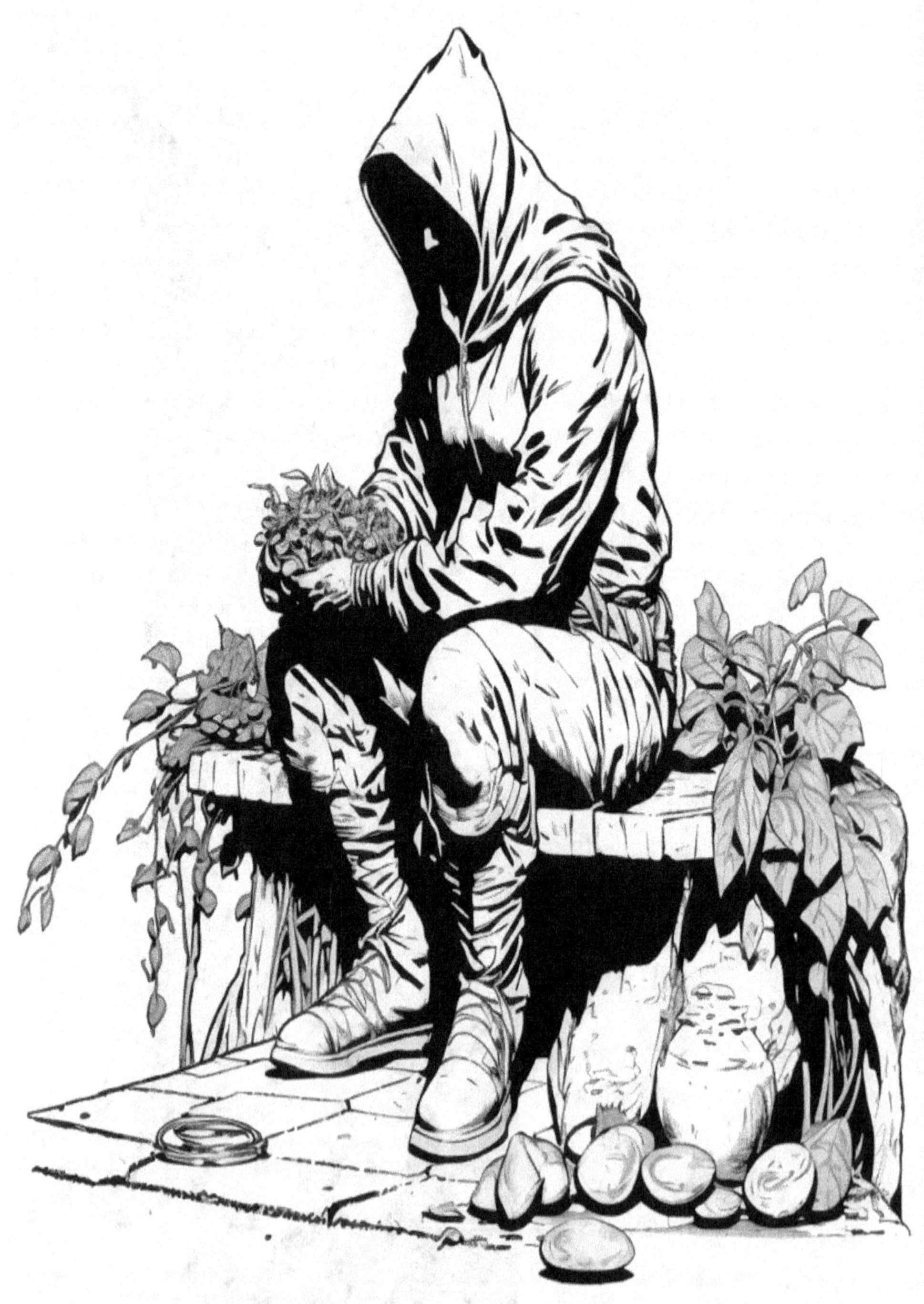

Microgreens are not only delicious, but they are also packed with nutrition. Here are some of the nutritional benefits of microgreens:

1. Vitamins: Microgreens are a great source of vitamins, including vitamin A, vitamin C, and vitamin K. These vitamins are essential for maintaining healthy skin, immune function, and bone health.

2. Antioxidants: Many varieties of microgreens are high in antioxidants, which help to protect against cellular damage caused by free radicals. Antioxidants can also help to reduce the risk of chronic diseases such as cancer and heart disease.

3. Minerals: Microgreens are a good source of minerals such as calcium, iron, and potassium. These minerals are essential for maintaining strong bones, healthy blood, and optimal nerve and muscle function.

4. Fiber: Microgreens are a good source of dietary fiber, which helps to promote digestive health and can help to reduce the risk of chronic diseases such as diabetes and heart disease.

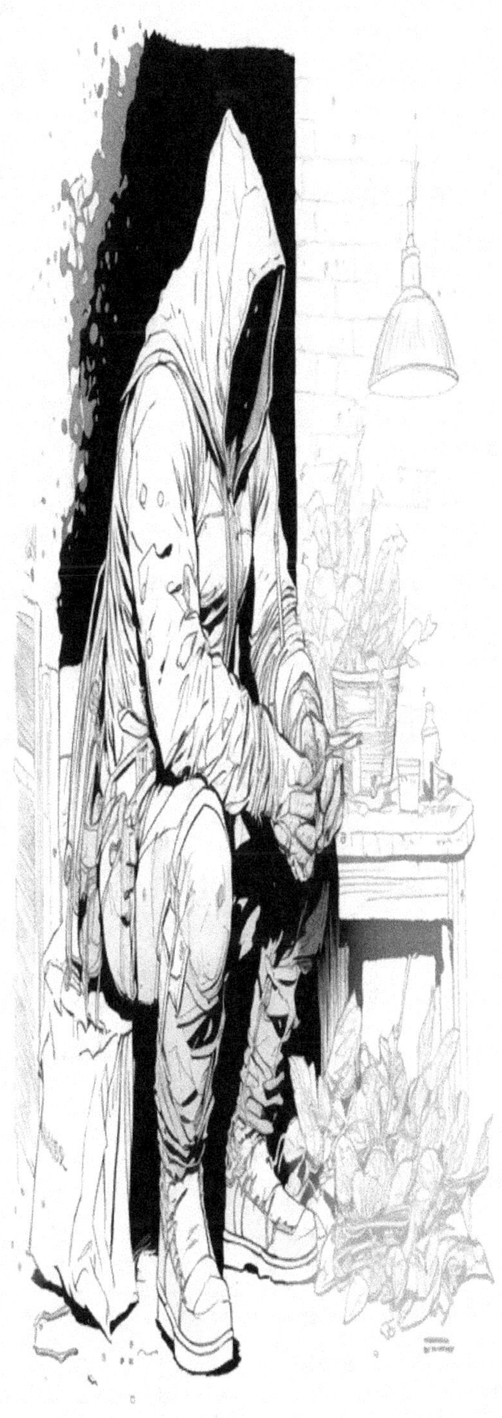

<u>**5.Protein:**</u> While microgreens are not a significant source of protein, they do contain some protein and can be a good addition to a plant-based diet.

By incorporating a variety of microgreens into your diet, you can enjoy their delicious flavors and reap the many nutritional benefits that they offer.

In the next chapter, we will discuss some creative ways to use microgreens in your cooking, including adding them to salads, sandwiches, and smoothies.

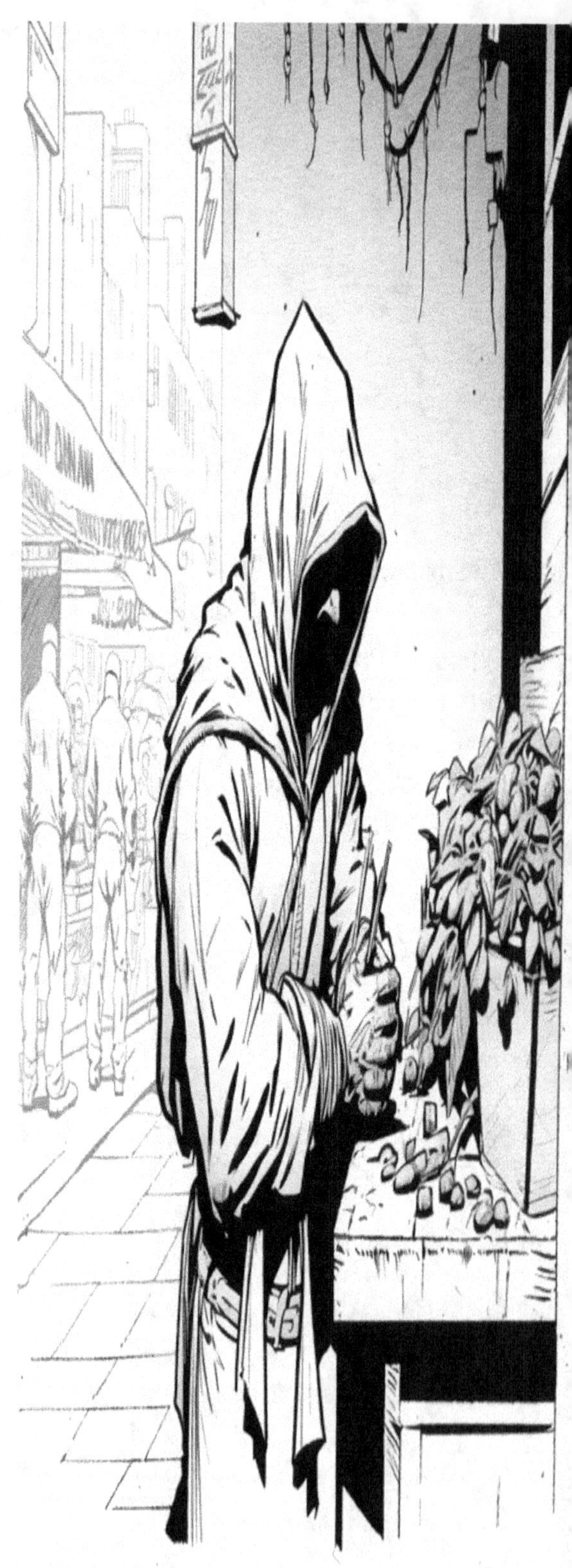

CHAPTER 12: CREATIVE WAYS TO USE MICROGREENS IN COOKING

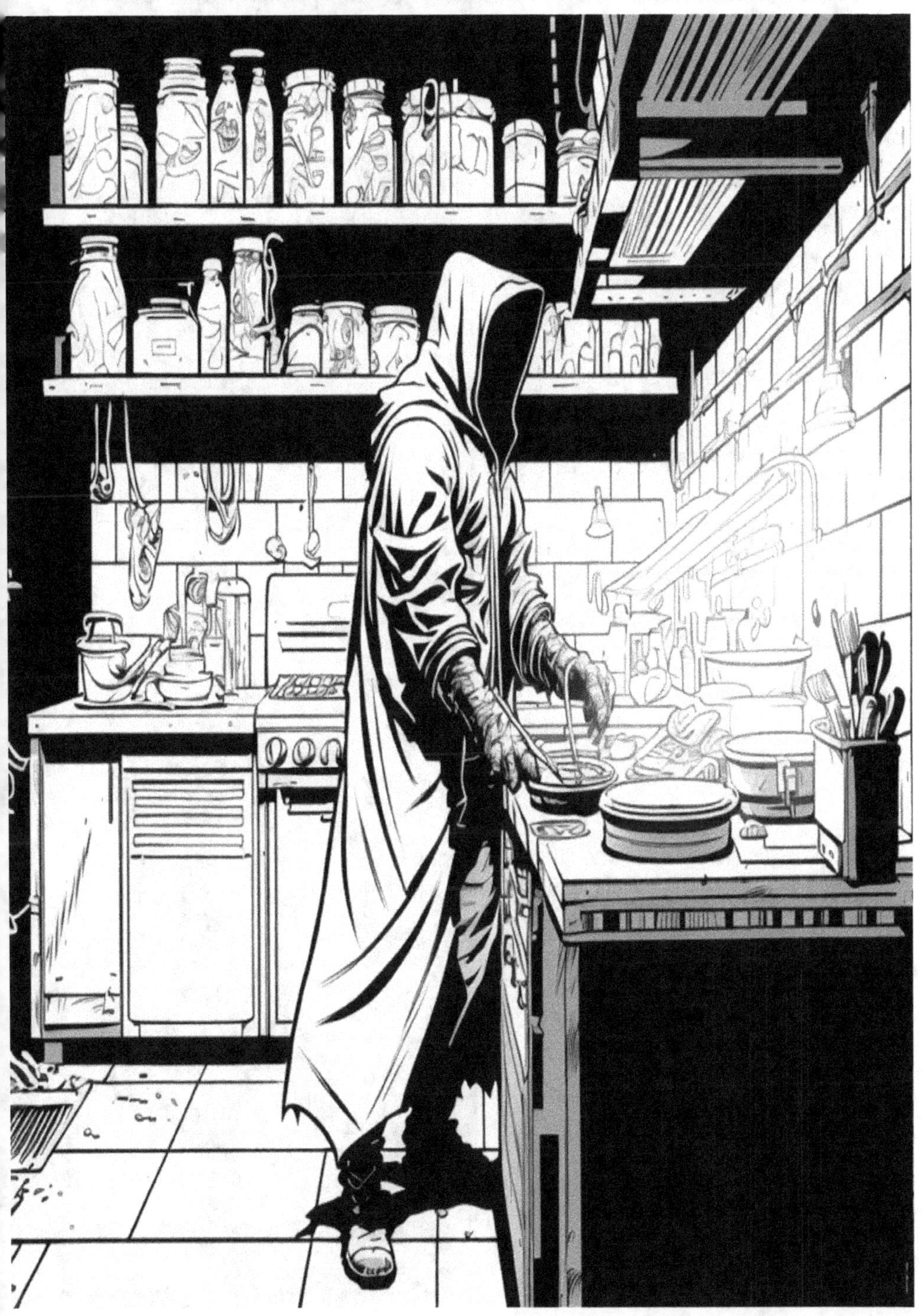

Microgreens can add a pop of color, flavor, and nutrition to a variety of dishes. Here are some creative ways to use microgreens in your cooking:

1.**Salads:** Add microgreens to your salads for an extra boost of flavor and nutrition. They pair well with other salad greens, as well as fruits, nuts, and cheeses.

2.**Sandwiches and Wraps:** Add microgreens to your sandwiches and wraps for a fresh crunch and a burst of flavor. They can also add some color and texture to your lunchtime favorites.

3.**Smoothies:** Add a handful of microgreens to your smoothies for an added dose of nutrition. They pair well with fruits such as berries, pineapple, and mango.

4.**Soups and Stews:** Top your soups and stews with microgreens for a colorful garnish and an extra boost of nutrients. They can also add some texture to your favorite comfort foods.

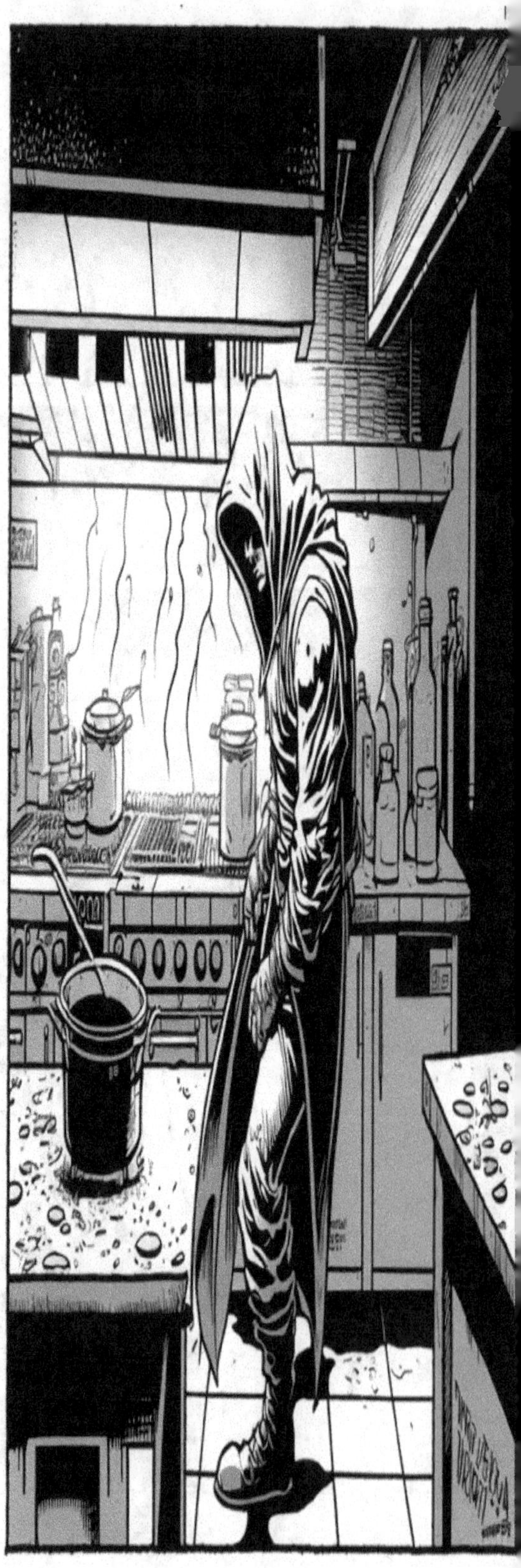

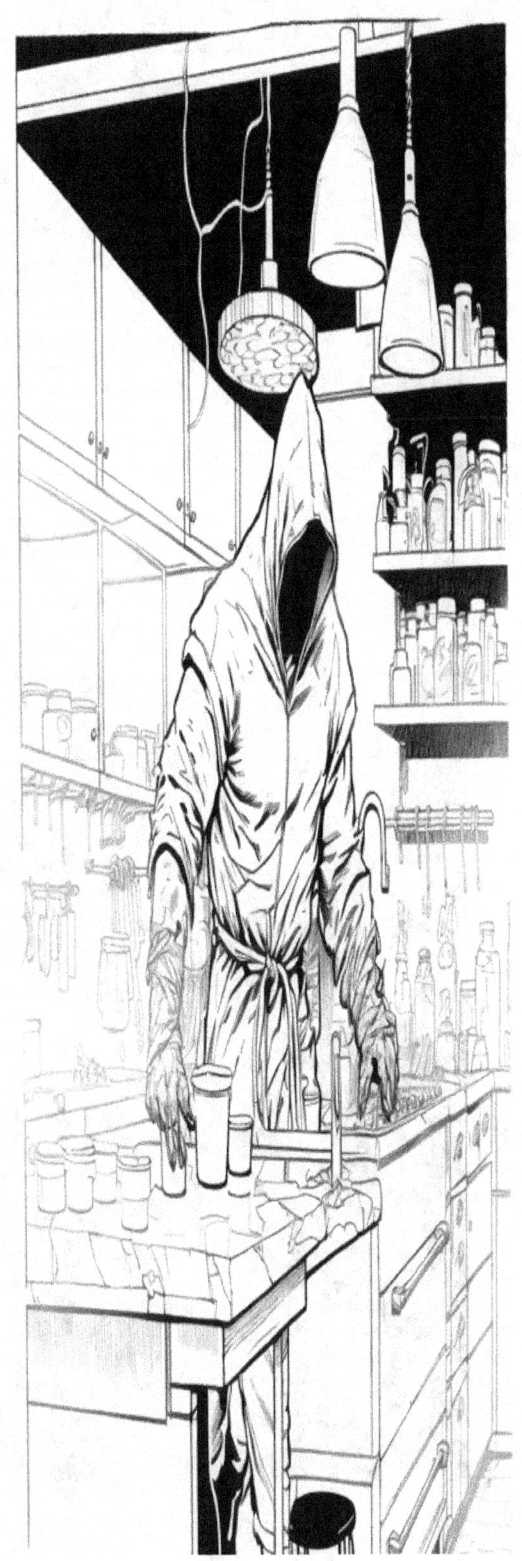

5.Pizza: Sprinkle microgreens over your homemade pizza for a fresh, gourmet twist. They pair well with toppings such as goat cheese, prosciutto, and roasted vegetables.

By incorporating microgreens into your cooking, you can enjoy their delicious flavors and reap the many nutritional benefits that they offer.

In the next chapter, we will discuss how to store and preserve your microgreens to ensure that they stay fresh and flavorful for as long as possible.

CHAPTER 13: STORING AND PRESERVING YOUR MICROGREENS

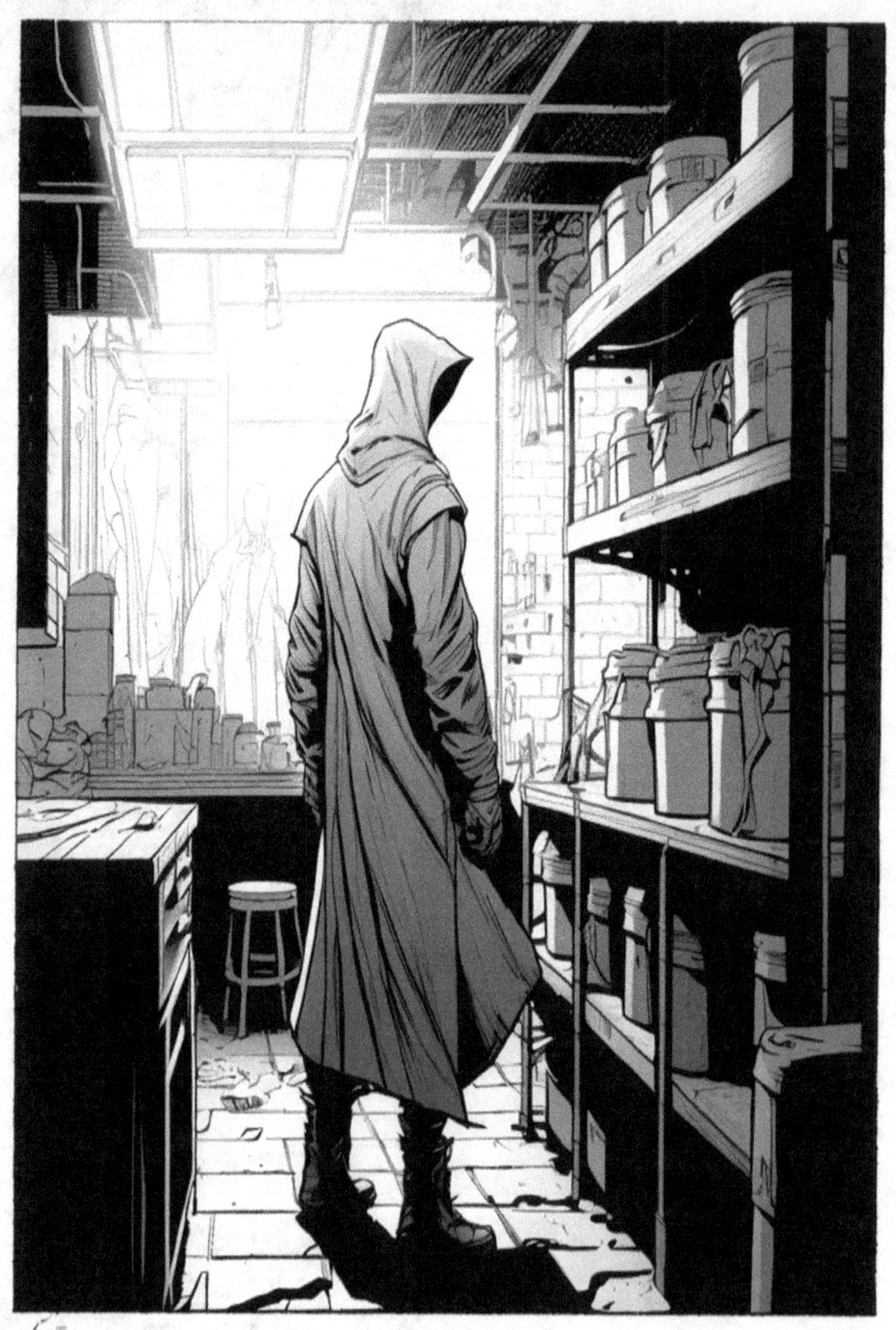

To get the most out of your microgreens, it's important to store and preserve them properly. Here are some tips for storing and preserving your microgreens:

1.**Store in the refrigerator:** Once you have harvested your microgreens, place them in a plastic bag or container and store them in the refrigerator. They should last for up to a week.

2.**Keep them dry:** Make sure that your microgreens are completely dry before storing them, as moisture can cause them to wilt or spoil.

3.**Don't wash them until ready to use:** Avoid washing your microgreens until you are ready to use them, as moisture can cause them to wilt and spoil more quickly.

4.**Freeze for later use:** If you have an abundance of microgreens, you can also freeze them for later use. Simply place them in a plastic bag or container and freeze. They should last for up to six months.

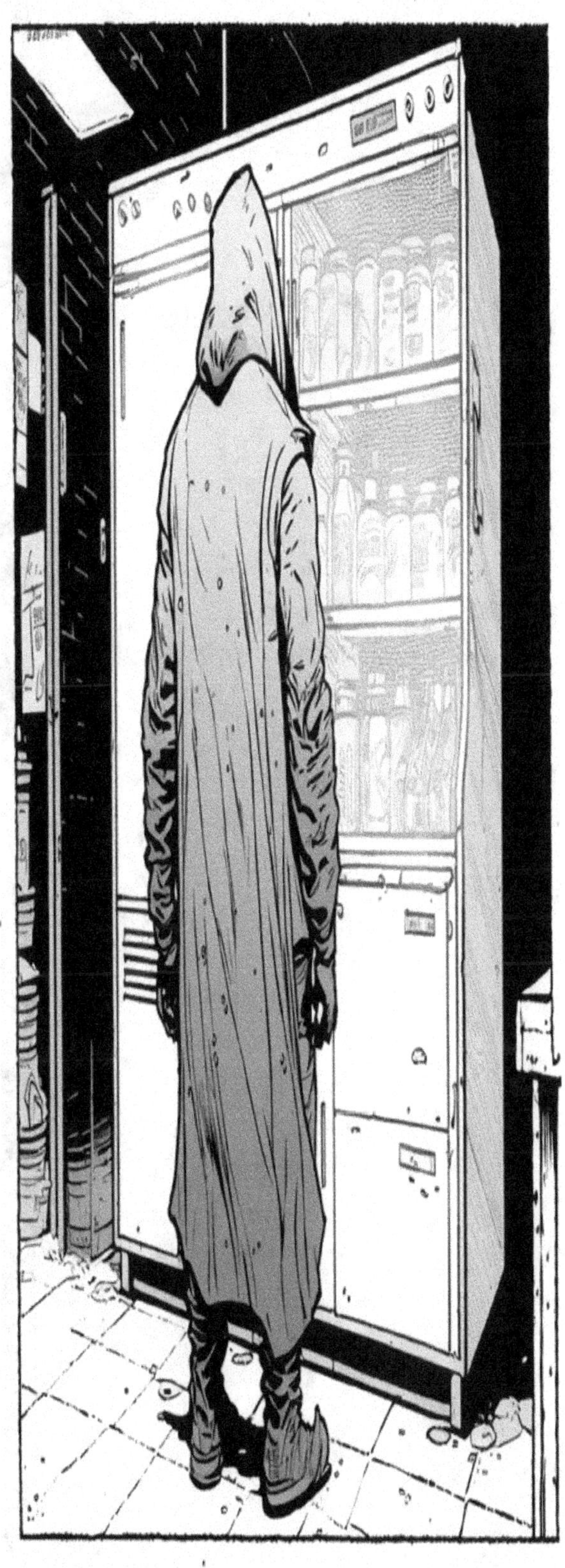

5. Dehydrate for longer storage:
If you want to store your microgreens for an extended period of time, you can also dehydrate them using a dehydrator. Once they are dehydrated, store them in an airtight container in a cool, dry place. They should last for up to a year.

By following these tips, you can ensure that your microgreens stay fresh and flavorful for as long as possible.

In the next chapter, we will discuss the environmental benefits of growing your own microgreens, including reducing your carbon footprint and supporting sustainable agriculture practices.

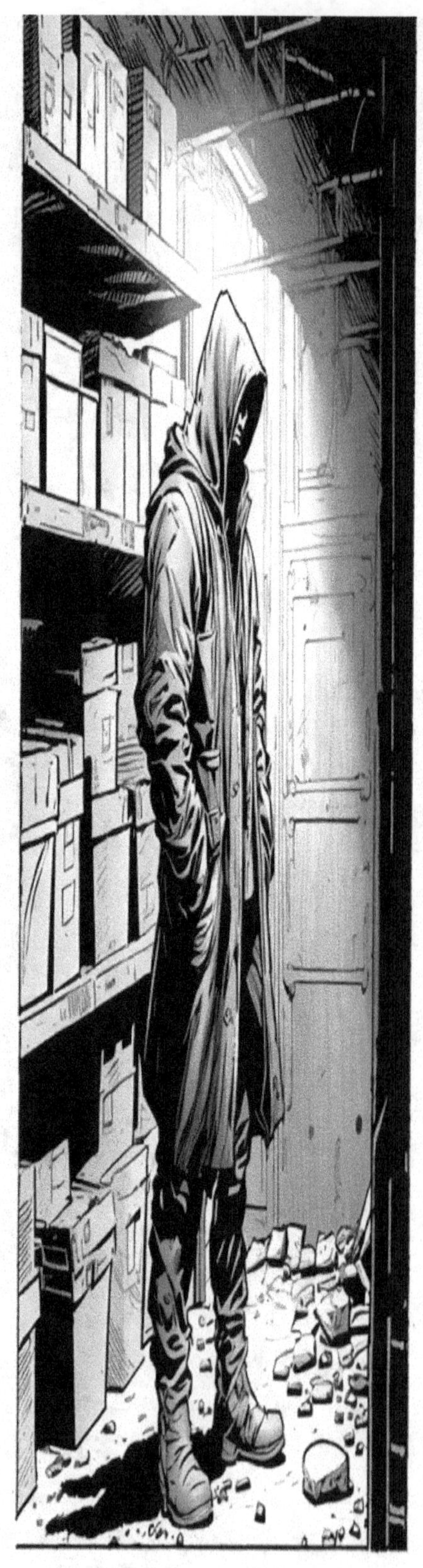

CHAPTER 14: ENVIRONMENTAL BENEFITS OF GROWING YOUR OWN MICROGREENS

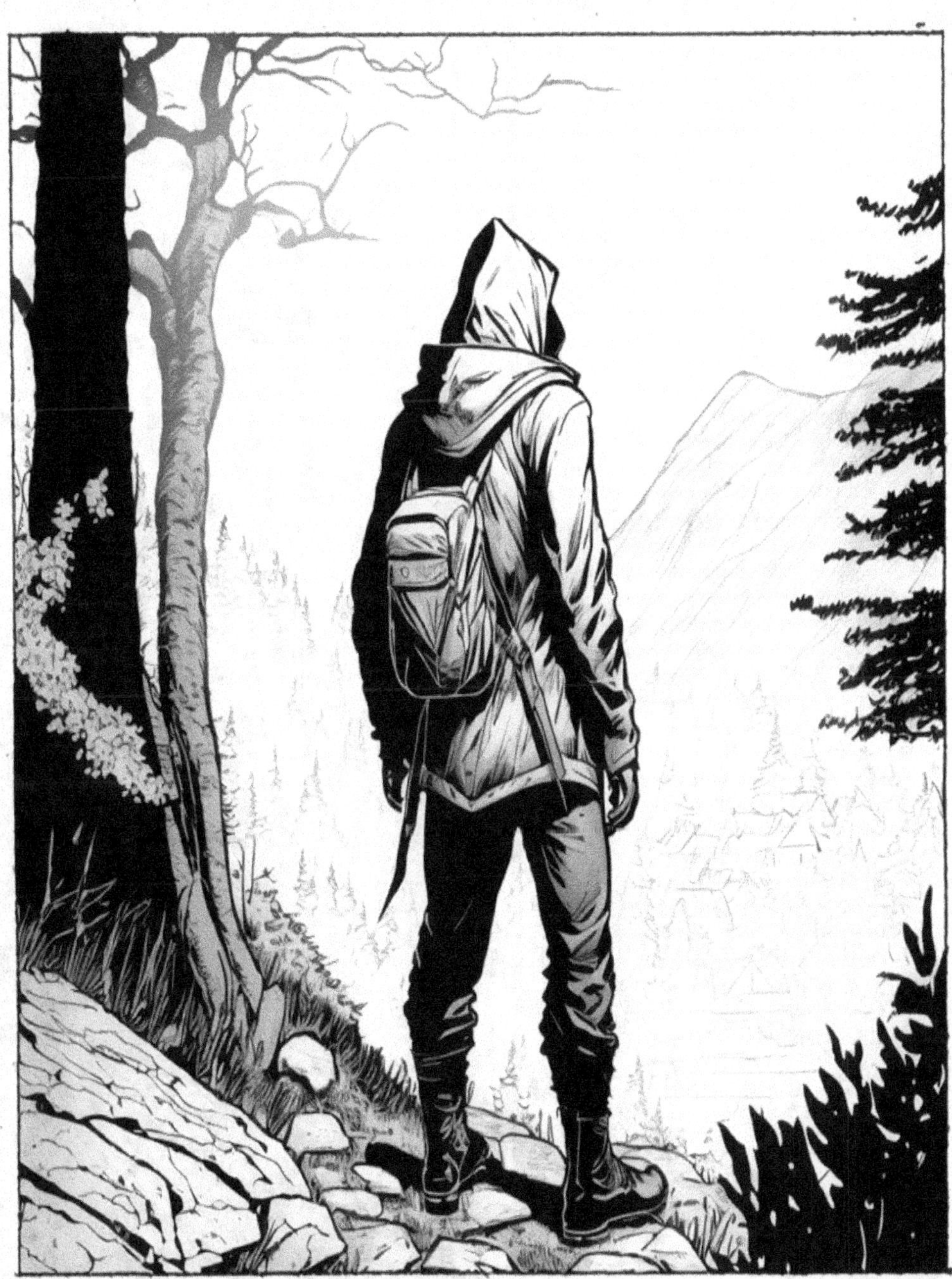

Growing your own microgreens not only provides you with delicious and nutritious food, but it also has many environmental benefits. Here are some of the ways that growing your own microgreens can benefit the environment:

1. **Reducing your carbon footprint:** When you grow your own microgreens, you reduce your carbon footprint by eliminating the need for transportation and packaging. This helps to reduce greenhouse gas emissions and supports a more sustainable food system.

2. **Saving water:** Microgreens require much less water to grow than traditional crops, making them a more water-efficient option for gardening.

3. **Supporting sustainable agriculture practices:** Growing your own microgreens allows you to support sustainable agriculture practices such as organic farming, reducing the use of pesticides and fertilizers, and promoting biodiversity.

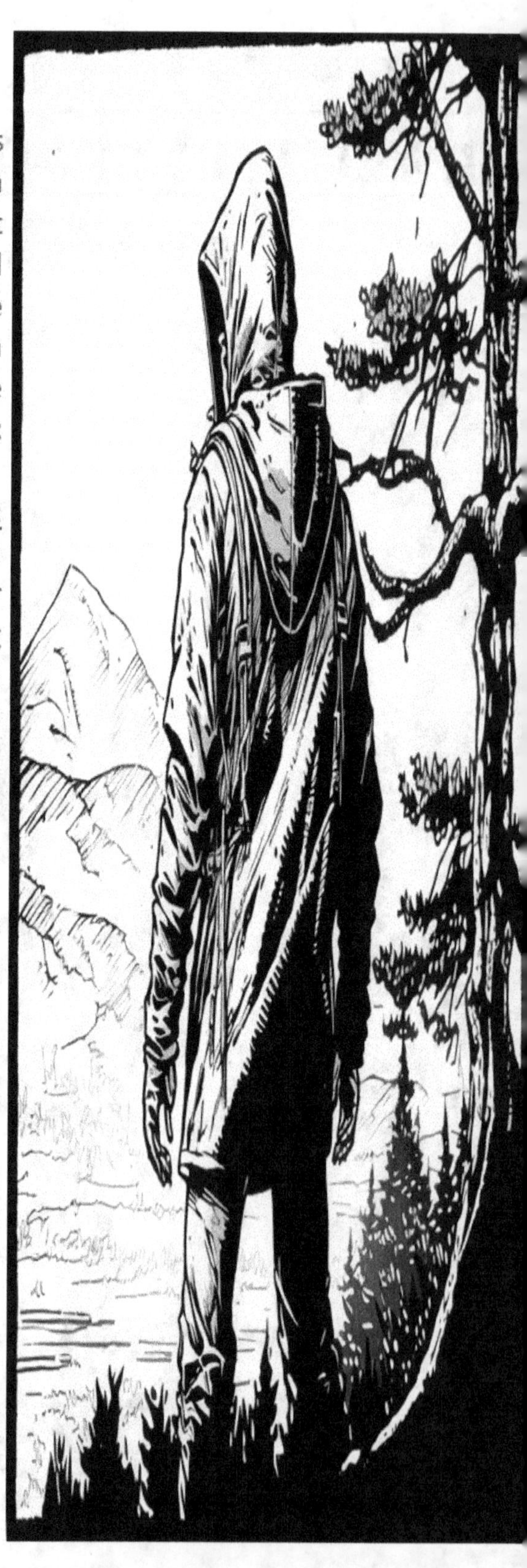

4.Composting: After harvesting your microgreens, you can compost the remaining plant matter to create nutrient-rich soil for your next crop.

5.Reusing containers: Growing microgreens allows you to reuse containers such as trays, pots, and jars, reducing waste and supporting a more circular economy.

By growing your own microgreens, you can take small steps towards a more sustainable and environmentally-friendly lifestyle. In the final chapter, we will provide some additional resources for growing microgreens, including books, online courses, and other helpful tools.

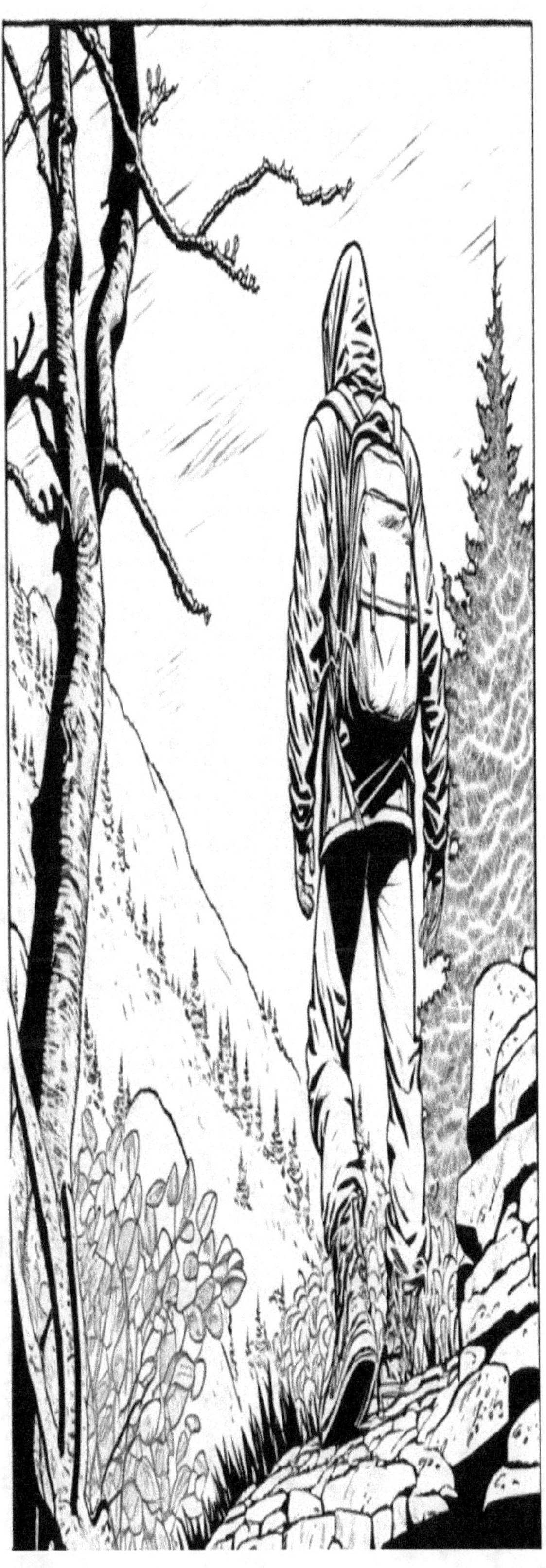

CHAPTER 15: ADDITIONAL RESOURCES FOR GROWING MICROGREENS

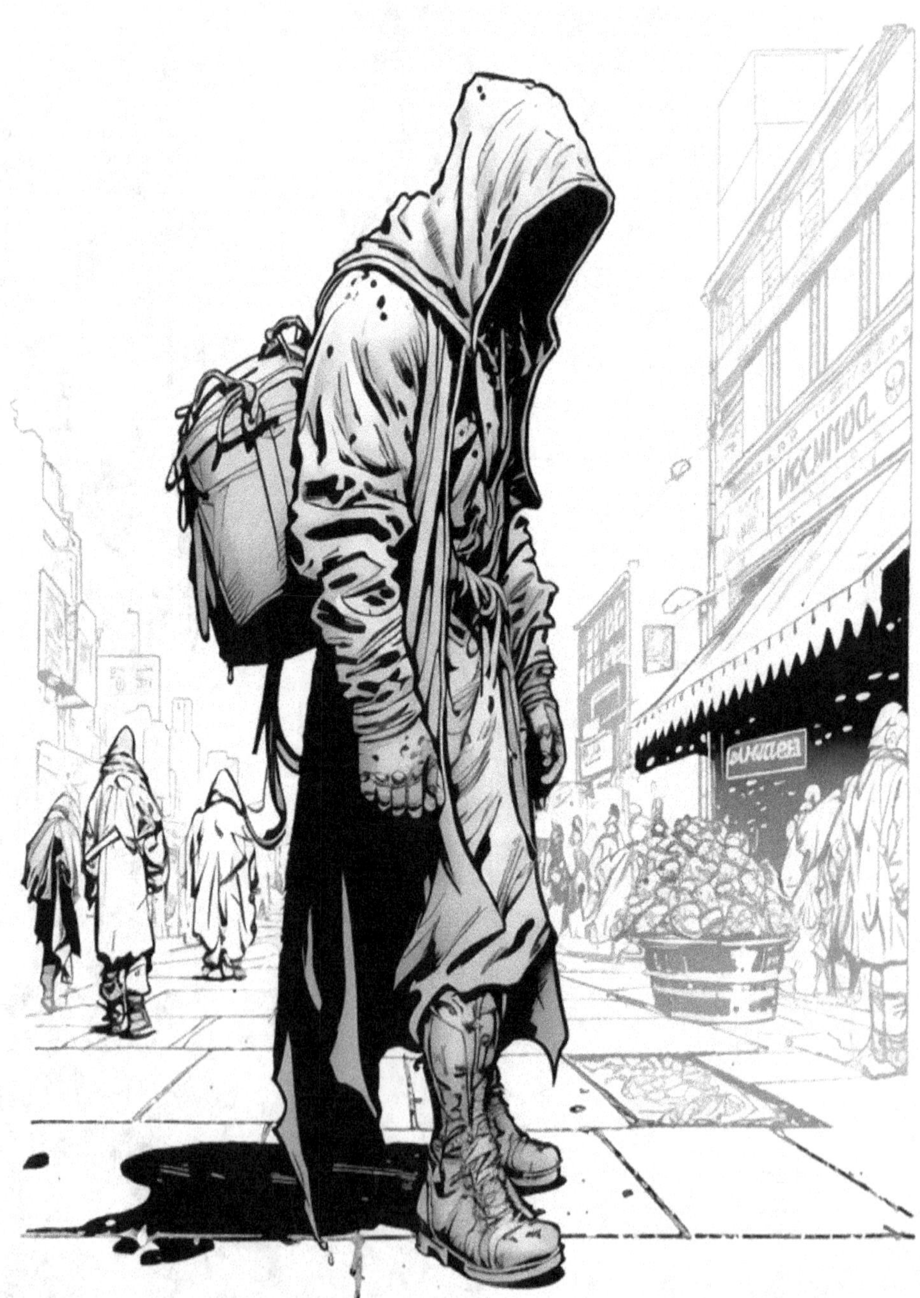

If you are interested in learning more about growing microgreens, there are many resources available to help you get started. Here are some additional resources for growing microgreens:

1.<u>Books:</u> There are many books available on the topic of microgreens, including "The Complete Guide to Growing and Using Microgreens" by Mark Mathew Braunstein and "Microgreens: How to Grow Nature's Own Superfood" by Fionna Hill.

2.<u>Online courses:</u> If you prefer to learn online, there are many courses available that can teach you the basics of growing microgreens. Udemy and Skillshare offer courses on growing microgreens, and there are also many free tutorials and videos available on YouTube.

3.<u>Seed suppliers:</u> There are many suppliers of microgreen seeds available online, including Johnny's Selected Seeds, True Leaf Market, and High Mowing Organic Seeds.

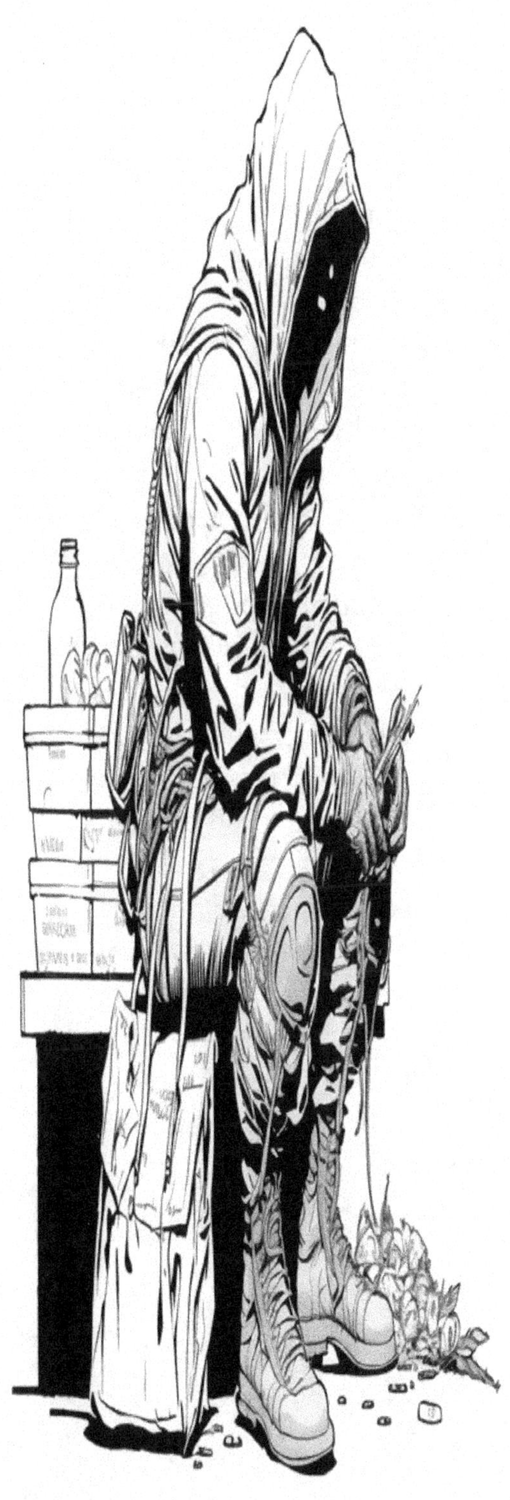

4.Microgreen kits: If you are just getting started with growing microgreens, there are many kits available that provide everything you need to get started. Some popular kits include the Hamama microgreen kit and the Click and Grow microgreen kit.

5.Local gardening groups: Joining a local gardening group or community can also provide valuable resources and support for growing microgreens. You can also share tips and ideas with other gardeners and get advice on how to troubleshoot any problems that you may encounter.

By utilizing these resources, you can become a successful and confident grower of microgreens. Happy growing!

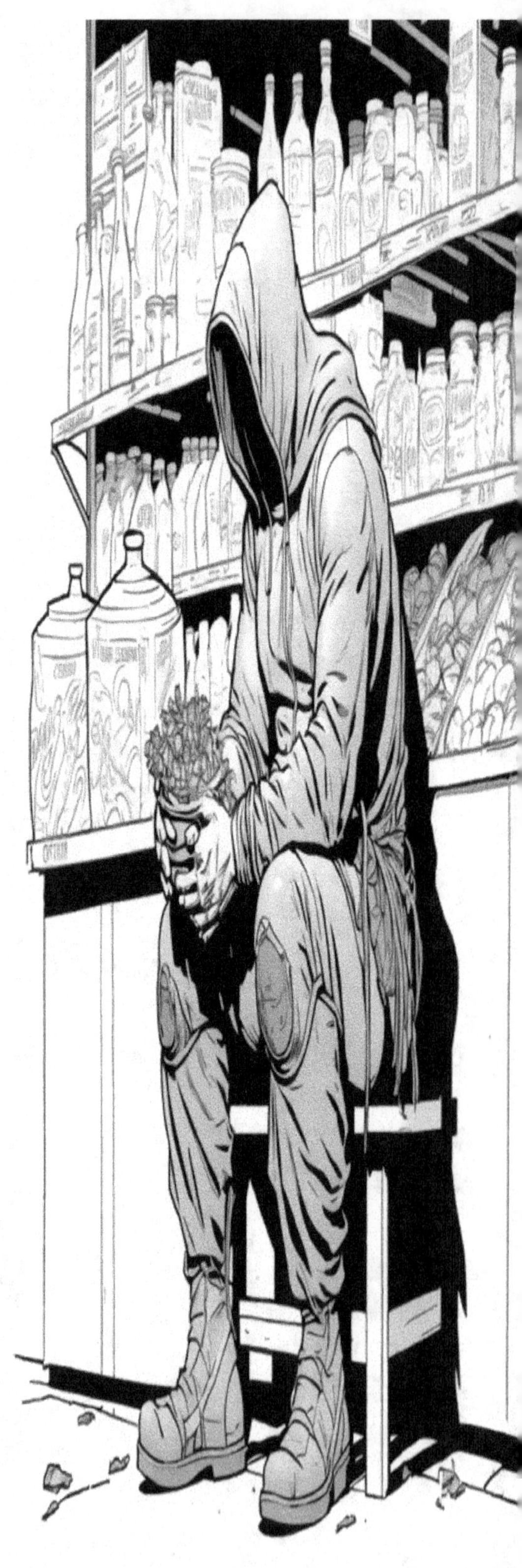

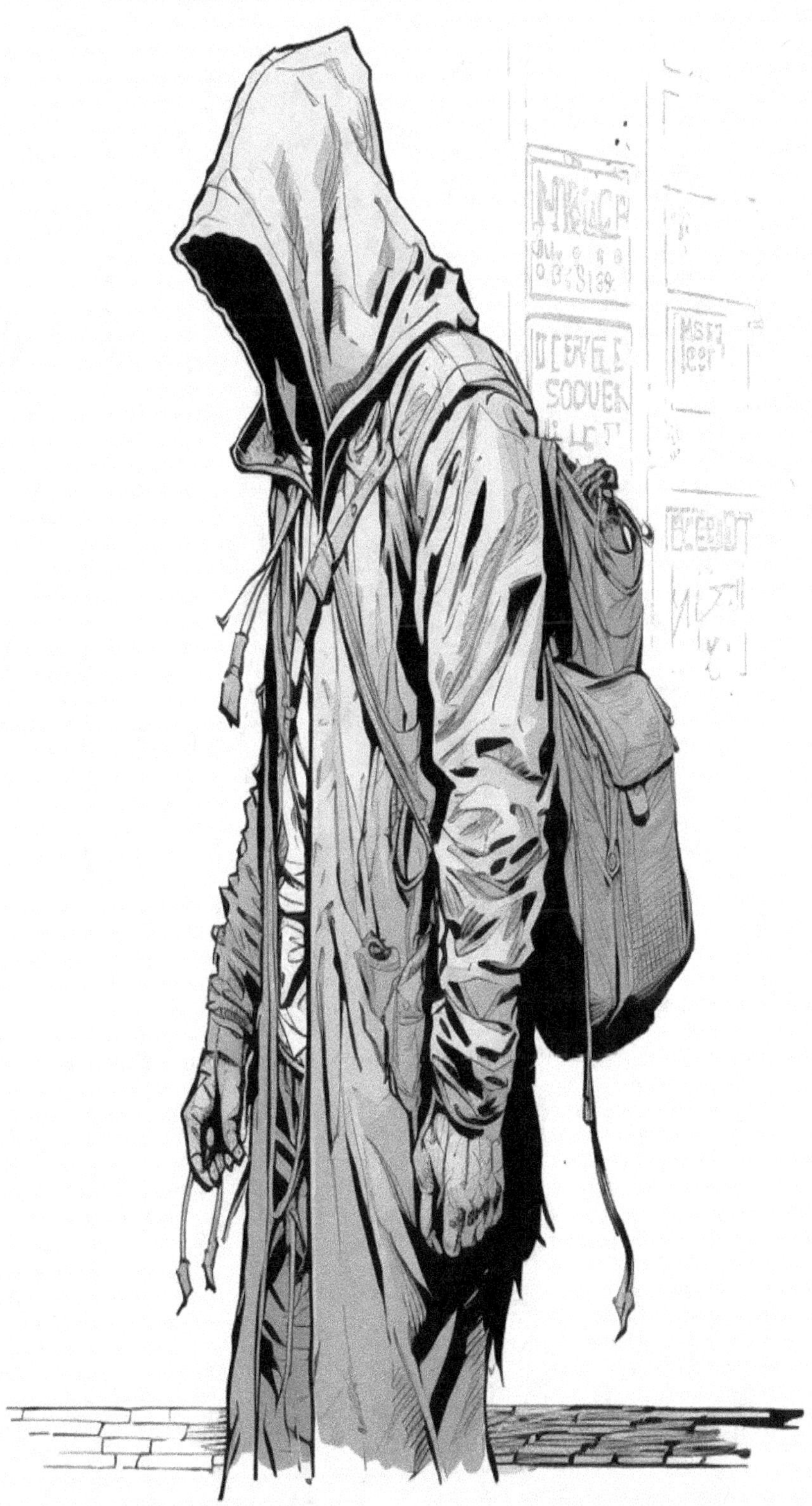